"Ask Dr. Flo"

150 Tips from Head to Toe
for Less Pain & Better Function

FLO BARBER-HANCOCK,
L.M.T., PH.D.

The information in this book supersedes all prior publications by this author on these topics.

Published by Richter Publishing LLC
www.richterpublishing.com

Book Cover Design: Jessie Alarcon

Editors: Marisa Beetz & Margarita Martinez

Book Formatting: Monica San Nicolas

ISBN-13: 978-1-945812-78-1

DISCLAIMER

DEDICATION

To my patients –
all of them, really—but especially to those who have
pushed me harder to learn more, do more, and share what
I have learned by writing and publishing this book.

CONTENTS

ACKNOWLEDGMENTS

First, I must acknowledge my husband, G. Dallas Hancock, D.C., Ph.D., who started me on my career in health care over two decades ago, and who has supported me in spirit and substance ever since.

I must also acknowledge the countless patients whose questions have prodded me to find better answers, and whose encouragement has been a strong incentive to get these "tips" into print. They've asked for my words in print—to take home, to share with others, and to ensure that what I have learned will still be available when I (eventually, maybe) retire.

I owe special thanks to Dave M. of Plant City, for constantly prodding me; to Pam M. of Tampa—I learned so much with you!; to Lisa G., one of my most challenging patients, who has had such an amazing recovery; to Mary Ann, for showing me what an indomitable spirit can achieve; to Frank and Barbara, who shared so much in this learning path, especially regarding glasses. Also to Janet W., for deepening my education in repetitive motion disorders; to Greg, for terrific humor in the face of physical challenges; to Skyler, who taught me so much about Lyme disease. To Sharon L-R, who first led me into understanding the link between repetitive motion and migraine headaches; and Martin, for giving me new insights into the links between vision, vision therapy, and somatic pain. So many other patients have contributed to the development of the "myofascial map" for my Facilitated Pathways Intervention and my growth as a therapist—this list could go on and on.

To all those patients and friends not mentioned by name, please know that I am so deeply grateful that you trusted me, allowed me to serve you, and contributed in ways you might never guess to my health care education and the writing of this book. And, to the special friends who offered to be my "beta-testers"—reading drafts to provide feedback because they have heard me talking about these topics for years—Lisa, Carrie, and Janet. And to numerous friends at my Suncoast Toastmasters International club, who have encouraged me and been models of success.

And very special thanks to my professional friends in other health care fields, who read chapters relevant to their expertise to "keep me honest": Lisa Landwirth, LCSW, and Heather Holt, Ph.D.

For the professional appearance, literary improvements, formatting, and cover design, I owe great thanks to the editors and other staff of Richter Publishing: Tara Richter, Margarita Martinez, Marisa Beetz, and Monica San Nicolas. Their assistance and support was vital in the preparation and completion of my manuscript and bringing it all together to this finished state, ready for publication.

INTRODUCTION

I've been in "helping" professions since my first job as a teenage babysitter. My bachelor's degree was in special education, and I spent 10 years teaching in elementary classrooms. From there, I segued into several other venues serving children and adults with special needs. I enjoyed all those positions, and raised two daughters along the way, but I had not found quite the right spot to capture my full attention—until I became reacquainted with Dr. G. Dallas Hancock.

One evening in 1992, we encountered each other in a social setting. We had been casual neighbors about 15 years earlier, and that chance meeting quickly blossomed into a friendship. Dinner conversations about careers and leisure interests identified our mutual interests in helping people feel better and function better. When he talked about how cranial techniques that he had developed could help children move better and read better, I was hooked. We began dating, and soon I was studying cranial anatomy and other aspects of health care. One year after that first encounter, I began assisting him with workshop preparations and clinical activities. By 1997, I was deeply involved in providing therapy under his supervision and thoroughly enjoying all aspects of our work. I wanted to have my own clinical practice, so I attended massage school in the evenings and became a licensed massage therapist in December of that year.

I have now been a clinician for over 20 years, treating people with recent and chronic pain. I use structural and functional cranial techniques to resolve many different musculoskeletal symptoms. My goal is to help each person get back to the activities they want to do, as quickly as possible. My practice is founded on holistic and functional concepts and evaluations of how the whole neuro-musculoskeletal system is working. I listen carefully to each patient's history of activities, traumas, and repetitive movements, so I have a better idea of factors that are underlying their pain. Biomechanical concepts of posture, balance, and movement are important aspects of how I assess a patient's symptoms and develop a treatment plan, and I always use testing of muscle function to confirm treatment results. My experiences and clinical findings led me to pursue a doctoral program, and my Ph.D. specialization in neurosensory rehabilitation. My dissertation was on the new type of neuro-myofascial (nerve-muscle-fascia) treatment that I developed through my clinical practice.

Each patient's evaluation includes an assessment of everyday items and activities that may be causing their pain or interfering with functional recovery from trauma. These items always include shoes, cell phones, and car seats, and usually glasses (we're in Florida—almost everyone has sunglasses); most seniors also have glasses for reading or distance.

These tips started out as conversations—answering questions that my patients often ask:

"What can I do to avoid having this problem and this pain come back?"

"What do I have to do so I don't have to keep spending time and money going back to my massage therapist/chiropractor/M.D., etc., every week?!"

"What can I do to take better care of myself between sessions with you?"

I've been giving my patients these tips for years. They're always grateful, but some say, "Oh, dear—I hope I can remember all that!" and a few have said, "You should write a book!" And at some point I realized that the short, scribbled notes I handed people were not enough—I *needed* to write a book to share the knowledge I had acquired through many years of clinical practice.

Dave, a frequent patient who started his own very successful business decades ago, kept prodding me: "When are you going to write that book?" Then Bonnie, another supportive friend and entrepreneur, recommended a book by Daniel Priestley. His concepts gave me another push and an idea on how to get started. I began in late 2014 by making a list of the twelve topics I discuss most frequently in the clinic. It has come together in fits and starts, in a life busy with many other activities, but the words have flowed easily. I *wanted* to write this book, not only for my patients, but for hundreds and thousands of other people who can use simple tips like these to make their bodies more comfortable, and life more enjoyable—at little or no cost.

1. SHOES (& SOCKS)

1) Worn down shoes

2) Athletic shoes

3) Flip-flops

4) Men's shoes

5) Women's shoes

6) Special-use shoes

7) Boots

8) Insoles

9) Outer soles

10) Cushioning in the soles

11) Spring-loaded heels

12) Arch supports

The nerves in our feet and ankles are one of the four major components of our balance mechanisms (the other three are in the head). Are the soles of your feet numb? If so, your brain is not getting important information that it needs to help you keep your balance. Have you had trouble with your equilibrium being a little off? Or taken a fall you think should not have happened? Foot numbness, and an absence of nerve input when you are standing, walking, climbing stairs, or running makes a fall more likely. And if you fall, it's a sure bet you will have pain or dysfunction that you did not have before.

Almost any kind of shoe can help or hinder muscle function and your body's daily movement demands. One style of shoe will never work for everyone. Whatever is between your feet and the ground has an effect on how your body balances. The feedback from your feet to your brain affects which muscles are "turned on" (working properly) or "turned off" (inhibited). That feedback affects your energy level and how well all of your muscles function when they're performing sports activities, gardening, or even cooking. Both bad feedback (from problems caused by your shoes) and lack of feedback (from your brain getting shortchanged because of numb nerves and fewer signals) can be significant contributors to muscle aches and pains that make your life less enjoyable.

Don't believe me? Try some of these tips—there's a dozen here to help your feet and body be more comfortable.

1)   Worn down soles. If any of your favorite shoes are worn down at the heels or on another part of the sole, have them repaired or **Pitch. Them. Out.** (New shoes cost less than therapists and doctor visits!)

2)   Athletic shoes. Find several different pairs of footwear, other than athletic shoes, for everyday wear. Unless you are involved in truly athletic activities all day, every day, owning just one specific kind of shoe is not a great idea for your health. And change is good not only for your feet and body, but also for your shoes. It lets the shoes fully dry from any perspiration and allows the uppers of the shoe to relax.

3) Flip-flops. Send ALL of your flip-flops and thong-type shoes on a permanent vacation—without you! (Well, okay—you can keep one pair, but only for the beach or pool.) Flip-flops are a really fast way to increase pain in the soles of your feet, your calves, lower back, upper back, and neck. Muscles in those areas get tighter and tighter with every step you take while wearing flip-flops. Headaches also tend to get worse. The stress that goes to your head can even reach your forehead or eyes!

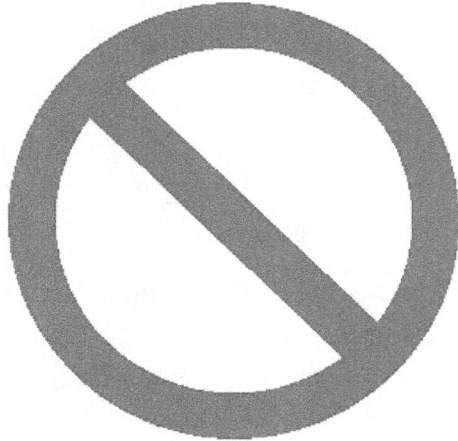

Why are flip-flops so bad? Because your toes have to clench with every step you take. That's the only way that (most) flip-flops stay on your feet. It's not just your toes that tighten—it's muscles in the arch of your foot, and your heel, and your Achilles tendon, and your calves … right on up to your head. Muscles get the message that you want them to be tight, so they get in that habit, and then you wonder why you hurt.

4) Men's shoes. If you shoe-shop in the men's aisles, whether you're buying/wearing slip-on shoes, or dress shoes with laces, be sure your shoes are not too narrow in the toe-box. If the toe area is too small, or too tight at the ball of your foot, it will have a constricting effect on many of your muscles. Whether you are presenting your ideas to a group, or just to one person you'd like to impress, you won't really be on your game if your shoes are too tight. Dress shoes, especially, can help you look great, but they also need to help you feel amazing, from head to toe.

5) Women's shoes. If you shoe-shop in the ladies' aisles, whether you're buying/wearing flats, pumps, sandals loafers, wedges, or heels:

Choose shoes that aren't too pointed and that have enough structure or straps to keep your heel in place and centered on the shoe. If your heel can slip to the side even a little, it will cause tension in your legs that can hurt all the way up to your head.

Really make an effort to avoid rigid platform shoes. If you'll be walking more than 100 yards or a city block in rigid soles, you're asking for pain. When shoes can't flex, neither can your feet. Flexing is necessary for normal, healthy movement, so your knees, hips, back, and neck are subjected to very unnatural stress in rigid soles. For dinner or a concert, you should be okay since you're mostly sitting; for a reception, cocktail party, or a trip to the mall—

save yourself some big regrets and choose shoes with a flexible sole.

6) Special-use shoes. Remember that some shoes are designed for a specific activity and not meant for everyday/any-surface wear. Special shoes for sports like soccer, golf, running, climbing, etc., may have a special place in your life, but limit them to those activities. Ditto for dance shoes and riding or cowboy boots. Five-finger "barefoot" style lightweight shoes, with individually enclosed toes, can be worn for a wide variety of activities, but they are still not an all-purpose shoe and aren't suitable for everybody.

7) Boots. Be sure any boots with laces (such as work boots and hiking boots) have the laces pulled nice and snug near your toes. Tightness there prevents your foot from sliding forward and banging your toe tips, which can cause calluses or blackened toenails from pressure bruising. The upper laces can be less tight.

8) Insoles. Insoles are where the sole of your foot contacts the shoe and carries your weight. The insole should be smooth, not bumpy. A raised area that provides arch support may be helpful for you. (See Tip #11.) Other raised areas, or hundreds of little bumps that may be marketed as good for cushioning or massaging the soles of your feet, can create problems. (See Tips #11 and #12.) Magnets in your shoes are also not healthy. (See Chapter 11, "Energy Fields.")

9) Outer soles. Choose outer soles that are suitable for the activities you will be doing and the surfaces/locations where you will be on your feet. Soles that are relatively smooth work fine for the home, office, or shopping. Soles that have ridges and grooves support more active foot movement and provide good traction when you are running or climbing outdoors, where footpaths and trails may have an irregular surface. Very flat soles provide the best grip on very smooth and potentially slippery surfaces, so deck shoes, court shoes, or medical-environment shoes are great if you're on vinyl, tile, hardwood, or marble floors. (Also see Tip #5.)

Shoes with rocker-style soles can create stress in your body. Whether or not such shoes are a good footwear choice is a very individual question. Rocker soles have been shown to be beneficial for the right person under the right conditions, but different brands and models have different attributes. They can reduce stress on some muscles and joints. On the other hand, they can increase stress on certain other muscles and joints, and they can even increase the likelihood of certain types of falls. So they're not "just another shoe" to pull off the shelf.

Rocker shoes come in models like "stable" or "unstable" and can considered a "training aid" since the very design requires muscles to work differently. Because they alter the way the foot rests when walking or standing, other parts of the body must compensate for the shift in weight distribution. For this reason, some people consider rocker shoes an orthotic, requiring a doctor's examination and recommendation.

At the very least, if you want to consider rocker-soled shoes, you should have an evaluation by a knowledgeable professional (not a shoe salesperson) to determine if rocker soles will benefit you, and if so, what model will work best given your health considerations, your body mechanics, and what your needs are for walking or running. The decision really comes down to your personal needs.

10) Cushioning in the soles. Gel or air-cushioned soles (and other overly cushiony components in the heels or soles of your shoes) can be a poor choice. When the sole of your shoe does not provide appropriate stability, the pressure nerves in your ankle may be overwhelmed by mixed messages. Your balance may be at risk if your ankle cannot provide the clear unambiguous information that your knees, hips, and brain need for good muscle control. An air-cushioned bounce house is fun for little kids who like to wobble and fall, but your shoes serve an entirely different purpose!

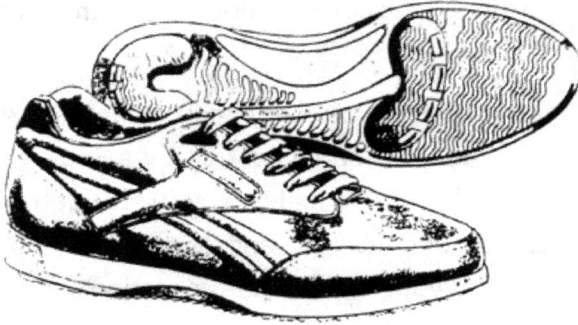

11) Spring-loaded heels. Putting a spring in your step? Not so fast, please! Avoid shoes with springs in the heels. They may (or may not) feel good at first, but they are likely to eventually cause extra stress for muscles and joints all over your body. Springs don't allow your foot and ankle to send dependable stability information to your brain. A little cushioning in the heel is okay, but when your heel strikes the ground, your brain needs unambiguous signals in order for your muscles to work most efficiently. Less effort = less stress = less pain. (See Tip #9.)

12) Arch Supports. The majority of orthotics are intended to provide support for the soles of the feet, particularly the arches. This discussion is limited to those types of orthotics. Tendons in the bottom of your feet lose strength and elasticity with age. As those strong cords get stretched out by time, gravity, and body weight, the arch flattens, providing less and less support. Those changes often result in the feet collapsing inward and ankles rolling toward each other. That puts an unhealthy stress on the knees, changing joint function as your knees also tip inward. These changes continue into the hips (more trouble can develop there) and from there, up the spine and to your neck and head.

Ideally, orthotics are personally designed for you, while you are seated, to fit your particular feet, and to bring your feet and ankles into the best possible position, which will reduce the stress on your body. But if you're standing when the orthotics are designed, then they will just keep you in the "collapsed" position that you're already in. They won't correct your foot alignment.

13) Socks. No discussion of shoes would be complete without mentioning socks. Remember this: not all socks are created equal! If you want your muscles to function better, or you just want to have fewer aches and pains, this tip is for you:

Socks that have a continuous band of extra elastic all around the foot—under the arch of the foot and on, up, and over the top of your foot—are putting more stress on your nerves and muscles. Don't buy them! The marketing people who write all those enticing words about "support'" and "energy" are not beta-testing the socks or assessing muscle function. Give such socks away, or throw them in the trash. Socks always cost less than therapy or doctors.

Why are these socks bad for you? Your feet have thousands of special nerves (proprioceptors) that respond to pressure. They help your brain decide which muscles to turn on or turn off in order to enable you to stand and walk, climb stairs, or run. You need good balance to do all these things. That band around the arch (on the bottom of your foot) and your instep (on the top of your foot) is stimulating too many nerves, and they're sending opposing messages to your brain: Lean left. No! Lean right. Lift up. No! Push down. Do all of these, right now!

You get the picture. Your brain is confused about what to do, so it turns many muscles into the off (inhibited) position. Every step you take then requires more energy. You'll tire faster; your balance won't be as good; your performance will suffer; and you may get neck pain, a backache, or a headache because of the increased muscle tension throughout your body. No socks are worth that!

2. SEATING

How often do you stop to think about how the chair, bench, or other thing you're sitting on is affecting you, adding to pain you already have, or changing the way your muscles function? Probably not often—until now. This chapter gives you tips on what seat to choose, and how to adjust the ones in your home, car, or workplace so you can be more comfortable.

14) Car seats. Do anything you can to adjust the seat position in your vehicle to make it more comfortable. It matters a lot to your aches and pains and your physical performance. First, get the back of your seat nearly vertical. If the back is slanted, it really creates a lot of extra stress on your neck muscles—and this stress will go all the way down your spine. (If you're tall and headroom is an issue, do the best you can.)

Second, get the seat pretty level across, from front to back, and from left to right. (See Tip #16 about chairs.) A level seat is extra important in your car because you have really limited options on changing your position. Additional physical stress is caused simply by being in a moving vehicle that has vibration, momentum, and changes in speed. The muscles throughout your body respond every time the vehicle slows down quickly or stops. If you're wide in the shoulders, the back of the chair (or car seat) may also create problems by bringing your shoulders inward. While driving, you're also keeping your eyes focused on the road, which adds to neck and shoulder tension.

Third, bring your seat forward enough for you to easily reach the gas pedal when driving. If your right leg has to reach to press down on the gas pedal, it increases the twist at your hips and can be a primary cause of sciatic pain, especially if you spend a lot of time behind the wheel. (Gas pedal extenders are available if you need one.)

Finally, make a habit of positioning your left leg and foot similar to the positioning of your right foot; that will help reduce the uneven twist at your hips. This is also true if you're a passenger.

15) Sofa, couch, or easy chair. Be sure to sit centered on the seat cushions of sofas, couches, and easy chairs—and don't cozy up to one arm of the chair. The seat supports are usually on each side and not all the way across. So, if you're closer to one edge of the seat, your hips are not equally supported. Therefore, they're not level—hello, twisted pelvis and achy body! You may also find yourself leaning over on the armrest, which can initiate another cascade of painful muscle compensations.

16) Sofa, couch, kitchen, and dining room chairs. Try to have your sofa and other seats at a height that lets your feet rest comfortably on the floor. If your feet can't rest comfortably flat on the floor, you may have just found a use for that neglected old phone book: footrest! If your legs are long and the chairs have wooden legs, consider adding the thickest nylon glides that you can find to the bottom of each chair leg. The goal is to have your thighs be parallel to the floor. Also, the seat needs to be pretty level across, from right to left, and from front to back. Flat seat cushions or pads are okay, but be wary of cushions that are button-tufted or otherwise lumpy.

17) Restaurants. In most restaurants, ask for a table rather than a booth. Booth seating is likely to be more uneven. If you're at all inclined to hip, back, or neck pain, a table with chairs will usually be a more comfortable choice, helping you to enjoy both your meal and the hours after it.

18) Barstools. Whether it's in a friendly kitchen or a public place you like to hang out, barstools are an invitation to bad posture. The challenge is for you to sit squarely on the seat. Don't have one hip half-on and half-off, with a leg dangling toward (or planted on) the floor. Especially if you combine a stressful way of sitting with twisting or leaning to participate in a conversation, or see a TV better, you won't be comfortable the next day! (Also see Tip #14, chairs.)

19) Recliners. Find a recliner that fits you all the way around: width (so you can sit centered and use the armrests without leaning), height (so your head and neck are comfortably supported), and length (so your legs and heels are supported).

Don't use a recliner instead of a bed. If you can't get comfortable in a good bed, you need to be seeing a health care provider who can identify and treat your medical or postural/structural (musculoskeletal) problems.

20) Sloped surfaces. This tip includes but is not limited to indoor seating. Avoid sitting on a chair, bench, swing, sofa, or rock that isn't level from left to right. Sitting on a sideways slope can often cause pain down one side of your body—but you may not know that until hours later. Be observant and smart up front: choose a seat that lets you face uphill or downhill—either is okay. You're asking for pain if you sit on a sideways-sloping surface for more than a few minutes, even if it's soft and inviting. You may encounter sloped seats in a room where chair legs are partially on a rug. Sloped surfaces are more frequently found on porches, in garages, or basements (which may have been converted to living spaces). Poolside decks, picnic table benches, garden benches, and some older homes with wooden floors may also provide unlevel seating.

21) Desk/office chairs. These seats need to be pretty level across, from right to left, and also from front to back, though there are ways to work around poor design. Seek out a chair, or modify one you have, to get a level seat surface that doesn't create musculoskeletal stress. Unless you have very slender hips, you may need to put a folded towel or a one-inch or two-inch cushion in the depressed center of the seat. If the sides of the seat are raised (as they usually are), that will roll your knees in toward each other, which contributes to pain in your low back or sacrum, and is also likely to stress your neck. (This is doubly true in vehicles: see car seats, Tip #14.) If you are wide in the shoulders, many car seats and some chair backs may create similar pain symptoms by bringing your shoulders inward.

22) Ball-chairs. Exercise balls (also called balance, fitness, or stability balls) have been adapted for office use. Yes, these "ball chairs" can improve your posture because you can't slouch. To stay upright on a fitness ball, your body has to make constant, small adjustments in muscle tension and weight distribution. Your muscles—especially those in your lower back—are doing the job done by a chair, namely, providing support and stability. So your back muscles spend hours being rigid. That constant tension and tightness in your back and legs is going all the way up to your neck and head, setting your body up for more back pain and less flexibility.

If you feel that you want to use an exercise ball chair, limit the number of hours you use it. Have a good chair (see Tip #20) and switch back and forth between the ball chair and a regular desk chair. My suggestion would be no more than two hours per day of non-continuous use of an exercise ball chair.

23) Bad seats. Bad seats are kind of like difficult relatives or coworkers—sometimes avoiding them is simply not an option. For those occasions, you just have to plan coping mechanisms to minimize your discomfort—and then leave ASAP! Visiting someone's home? Instead of sitting on an obviously lumpy or way-too-deep-and-soft-couch, ask to use a kitchen, dining, or folding-type chair, or almost any type of stool or bench. Tell the host you have a problem with your back. Even 15 minutes in an overstuffed sofa could have your back screaming all night. That is honestly "your back being a problem"!

At public events, carry a hand towel that can be folded as needed to make a theater seat or outdoor bench more

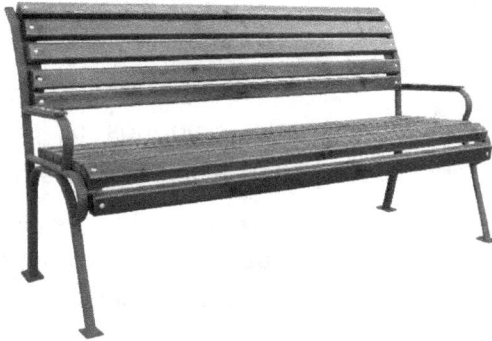

level. Try to sit somewhere that you can easily get up and stand or walk around now and then, so you're not sitting in one position too long without giving your muscles a stress break.

24) Bleachers, benches, and other hard seats. (Yes, this may include the seating in a religious center.) An easily portable seat that can provide some back support is worth the cost and effort. You can even take these devices where other people might not—for example, to a doctor's office. Sometimes the seats in such places are really not comfortable, and you may be sitting there a rather long time. It's your body and your life. If it means you'll get a better night's sleep or have less pain the next day, just do it. Be good to your body. Take along something that will make hard, soft, or poorly designed seats less stressful on your muscles and joints.

25) Anywhere. Try to avoid extended periods of sitting, especially if you tend to get neck or back pain. This includes meetings and when traveling by car, airplane, bus, cruise ship, or anything else. Get up and walk around! Up and down the aisle, stairs, or to the back of the room. Even stand in the back of a meeting room for a bit. Your vertebrae actually have more pounds of pressure per square inch when sitting than when you're standing. Pain tends to be reduced when you stand and walk around because movement activates many muscles, which improves the flow of blood and lymph in your legs and back. (Lymph is the clear liquid that fills a blister and creates swelling around a sprained joint. It flows through and between all of our cells, and it is moved by the action of muscles.)

3. VISION, BALANCE, & GLASSES

Our eyes usually adapt so quickly to our visual needs that we are seldom aware how many of our muscles are working in coordination with our eyes. How well your eyes are working can have a significant effect on your ability not only to see, but also on balance, dizziness, and vertigo. Here are three bits of information that will help you understand why eye function affects not just your neck, but also your whole body. Whether your vision is 20/20 or you have some vision problems, read on ...

➢ Vision and eye function are an important part of our four-part balancing system. The role of the eyes in balance is called the "ocular righting reflex."

➢ The eyes work in very close coordination with the little semicircular canals (fluid chambers) located in the ear that help keep you balanced against gravity. This function is called the "vestibular righting mechanism."

➢ The movement of each eyeball is controlled by six muscles. Five of these six muscles attach at the back of the eye socket to a single bone (the sphenoid) that goes behind your eyes, from one end of your eyebrows to the other.

➢ The subtle movements of the sphenoid and its thin, flexible, bony "wings" on each side relate a lot to the front part of your shoulders. Therefore, shoulder problems and eye/vision problems are sometimes related in very unexpected ways.

26) Vision and positions. It doesn't matter how good (or bad) your vision is—lying down to watch TV puts stress on your eye muscles that can create real problems in the function of other muscles, starting with your shoulders. Find a better position, where both of your eyes are in the same horizontal plane as the TV, or whatever you're looking at. If you're spending screen time with a laptop or other electronic screen (or any kind of print on paper, for that matter) the same rule applies. Your two eyes and the horizontal edges of the screen (or the print) need to be parallel to each other. (See also phones, Tip #42.)

27) Sunglasses. Whether your sunglasses are prescription or not, it's really best to avoid the wraparound styles that curve around the sides of your face. Seek out styles that have a boxier shape. A curved lens distorts what you're seeing, creating significant stress in your eye muscles, which then affects muscles in your face, neck, shoulders, and beyond. Bright sun, glare, hours outside, or sensitive eyes require good, all-around protection—but make a choice that's good for the rest of your body, and you may save yourself from a headache too.

It's also important to adjust the brightness of the screen on any electronic device to where it feels comfortable for your eyes. (See phones, Tip #41.)

28) Drugstore reading glasses. Glasses that are the wrong size for your face can cause muscle aches, pain, and muscle weakness where you least expect it. It's important to get glasses that properly fit your eyes and your face. Granted, inexpensive drugstore "magnifiers" can be a quick and easy fix if your eyes only need a little help now and then—like a menu in dim light or tiny print on a package label. But if you find yourself reading the paper, a report, or a book with them? You really need to get a pair that fits you.

The magnifying centers of the lenses need to match the center-points of your eyes: the distance between your pupils. (This is the same reason that the center hinge on good binoculars allows you to bring the eyepieces closer together for a narrower face or spread them wider for a larger face.) The long "temple" pieces of the glasses that rest on your ears need to be long enough to reach behind your ears comfortably, but not too long because then the glasses will slide down your nose. The bridge of the glasses needs to sit comfortably on your nose and not slide down. Adjustable pads are better than solid molded plastic.

29) Prescription lenses. Quality and service matter for prescription lenses. Choose the best quality that you can afford. Keep in mind that chain and franchise vision centers generally rely on volume and lots of advertising. A local optometrist (an excellent choice for routine eye care) will depend much more on word-of-mouth and referrals from satisfied patients. They're also likely to have the same staff for a longer time, so they can get to know you. (Check our website, www.HancockClinic.com, for a FREE download: "Tips for a Good Vision Exam.")

30) Know your types of eyeglass lenses:

➤ **Single lens**—only one kind of visual correction with no complicating factors.

➤ **Bifocals**—your eyes need help for two kinds of visual tasks, often close work and distance vision. The corrections can be separated so that you know when your eyes move from close to distance (bifocals) or have an area of continuous change (progressive lenses). Your eyes may prefer one type or the other.

➢ **Trifocals**—your eyes need help for three kinds of visual tasks: close work, a "middle range" for computer or conversational vision, and distance vision. The separation on the lenses can be continuous (progressive), linear, or a newer "office" style of the three corrective areas. The "office" style seems to avoid some of the focusing difficulties that can occur with progressive lenses. Newer ways of grinding these lenses (the "computer-distance" in the middle is narrower) make these a good choice for many people. You need to be able to have an informative conversation with your eye care professional about which types of lenses will be best suited to your visual needs and daily activity habits. Don't let yourself be talked into a style by high-pressure sales tactics.

31) Contact lenses. These are not suitable for everybody. If they're a reasonable choice for you, then go for it. They're the best (non-surgical) corrective lenses from a body-function standpoint. Because the lenses float on the fluid surface of your eyeball, they are always the correct distance from your eye. If they get off-center, you will usually know it immediately, and you can correct the problem yourself by re-centering the lens right away; no need to go to an optical center. (See Tip #34.) Note: Certain blue tints in corrective lenses may create a problem for vision or sleep, especially in older patients.

32) Frames. Eyeglass frames come in an incredible array of shapes, colors, and types. You will usually be wearing the frames for several years, so be sure to choose a frame that will be comfortable for the long term.

> **Molded plastic frames** have a molded bridge that just sits on your nose. These are often the cheapest type of eyeglass, but this type of frame is also used in some higher-priced styles. The lack of any way to adjust this single-piece bridge to the shape of your nose gives this type of frame a tendency to slide down your nose. When that happens, the glasses are no longer in correct alignment to your eyes, so your eye muscles have to strain, which then creates stress or pain in other muscles of your body. The part that rests on your ear (or wraps behind it) is also frequently quite rigid and is often limited in its ability to be shaped for a more secure fit.

> **Rigid metal rims**, with hinges at the corners and adjustable pads at the bridge of your nose, tend to be the best type of eyeglass frame for your body. Since those little pads can be adjusted to fit your nose, they tend to stay in place better. The metal frame may or may not go all the way around the lens. Either way, if you treat your glasses with reasonable respect, these frames can hold good alignment with your eyes for many months. This type of frame is also likely to be more adjustable at your ears, further ensuring a stable fit that minimizes the possibility of eyestrain from misalignment.

> **Flexible metal frames** (often titanium) are very lightweight, flexible, and sometimes marketed as "indestructible." Unfortunately, the lightness and flexibility also mean that they're too light and too flexible to stay in one place on your face. Therefore they don't usually do a good job of providing the stability that is necessary to keep the lenses in correct alignment with your eyes. These frames tend to be the most expensive, but they also seem to be the type that creates the most eye and muscle discomfort.

33) Styles. The style you choose will be most flattering if it is appropriate to the size and shape of your face. That said, larger lenses tend to be a better choice for glasses that are bifocal or trifocal; each area of correction needs to be large enough for your eyes to focus easily.

Smaller lenses may be fine if you only need a single correction, especially if they're for close work, like reading or computer use. For distance vision, however, larger lenses are a better choice. You'll need to turn your head less frequently, so there will be less stress on your neck muscles.

Small "readers" that perch toward the tip of your nose may be an option if you only need correction for close work and like to look at the rest of the world without glasses — but be sure they're designed to be worn that way.

34) Fit. Avoid frames that aren't selected or assembled specifically for your face (the side pieces are usually ordered separately to get a correct fit). That means care needs to be taken to get the proper fit for the width of your face and the spacing of your eyes. It also means having a "temple" piece (which reaches back to rest on your ears) that is the correct length for your head. If the frame you prefer can't be ordered in your size, then choose a different frame, or go to another vision center to find more variety and better choices.

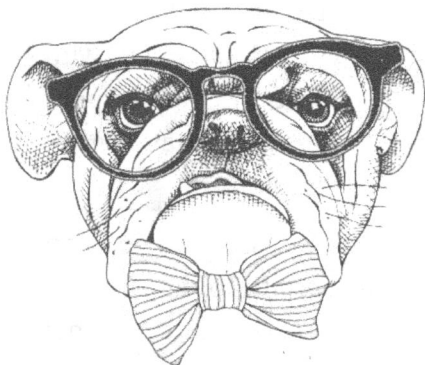

35) Alignment. A pair of glasses not properly fitted and aligned on your face is one of the most common self-induced causes of pain in people who otherwise seldom have eyestrain or headaches. Misalignment also causes a lot of other pain because very few people make the connection between poor alignment of their glasses and joint or muscle pain. This problem is usually one of the easiest and cheapest to correct.

> If your glasses are even slightly crooked, your body may be more doggone unhappy than this poor guy

The business where you bought your glasses should adjust the frames at no charge as often as needed. Even glasses that are treated gently get out of alignment over months of wear. If you take your glasses off with one hand, they will get out of alignment more quickly (so take them off with two hands, or at least by gripping them near the center). If they slide down your nose, the focal length changes, putting stress on your eyes and body. If the frames get even slightly twisted, that creates a different pattern of stress throughout your body. If one lens is higher than the other, or more forward (farther from your eye) than the other, different eye stress occurs, and both of these misalignments can create a lot of discomfort in your body.

In short—get your glasses aligned! And if you're having headaches, or your body hurts for no apparent reason, get your glasses aligned first and see if you hurt less. It's a step in the right direction for your vision and your muscles—and usually free.

36) Goggles, shields, and other protective eyewear. Some sports and workplace environments require protective eyewear. To whatever extent possible, choose goggles or shields that aren't too curved. Those with a bend at the corners are a better choice. Any eye protection (including sunglasses) that is shaped in a continuous curve creates stress in your eye muscles—and in your body muscles—because of the distortion that occurs as result of the curve. Your brain may be able to correct for the visual distortion so objects appear normal, but your eyes and body will still have to put up with the muscle stress that is occurring.

37) Windshields (yes, really!) This is worth checking if you spend a lot of time in the front seat of a vehicle and experience visual stress or body stress on long drives. This is especially true if you're the person who is driving. Brightness is also a visual stress. Such visual stress can also translate into body stress, so use sunglasses if it's a bright day, and try changing the position and angle of your seat to reduce visual and postural stress. Another possible problem is not common, but I have evaluated patients for whom the curve of the windshield appeared to create visual stress. In such cases, adjusting your seat position can be helpful.

4. PHONES—DUMB & SMART/OTHER SMALL SCREENS

Cellular phones have become a ubiquitous part of our modern lives. Each year brings better quality, more features, and an increased capacity for tasks of every sort. This trend seems likely to continue for the indefinite future, so we really all need to be paying more attention to how we use these devices, and how we can minimize their negative effects on our bodies and our lives. Whether you're buying your first electronic device or replacing one you already have—read on …

38) Visual concerns. A typical cell phone or smartwatch requires the use of near vision focused on a very small screen. This may not create a problem for adults whose eyes already have an established focal length (as "nearsighted" or "farsighted"). Children's eyes, however, are still developing. There is some research that indicates that too much use of cell phones, tablets, and similar electronic devices with small screens may contribute to the development of nearsightedness in children. Being outside in fresh air and sunlight protects growing eyes more than physical activity indoors. It's more difficult for young eyes to focus on an image, which causes the eye to change shape in order to see clearly. As more research becomes available, it's a good idea to seek up-to-date information on the effect of screen time on eye development.

39) Screen and image size. Enlarge the words or images on the screen so you can read or see more easily. The size of the visual display is an obvious consideration, whether your phone is a dumb phone or a smartphone, or even if you're using a larger screen such as a reader, tablet, or notepad. If your eyes are straining, your neck, shoulders, and other muscles may also become painful. The image size will affect how close you need to be.

40) Electromagnetic fields. (See also Chapter 11.) Electromagnetic fields (EMF) affect muscles. The signals from any device are more intense when sending or receiving. If reception or connection is poor due to distance from a cell phone tower (or a low battery charge in your device), this can increase the amount of electromagnetic activity. If your device has to work harder, then the EMFs are stronger, and that means they have a greater effect on your body. (See Tip #40.) If you frequently wear, carry, or use a device without enough EMF shielding, you may develop pain in a hand, hip, shoulder, leg or somewhere else as a direct result of EMF stimulation. The instruction booklet that comes with your phone, printed or online, is likely to carry a warning about EMFs. The warning message that accompanied my most recent phone was on page 23 in very small print.

41) Shielding. A case for safety. The quality of the case for your device will determine how much the electromagnetic field is affecting your body. Well-designed cases (such as OtterBox© or Bullet-Proof©) offer good EMF protection. This is your body (or maybe that of your child or older parents) and your health is important to protect. These shielding tips apply not only to your phone but also to your laptop computer and electronic reader. A cancerous response to EMFs is not out of the question if an electronic device is close to or touching the body for long periods of time.

42) Brightness. Adjust the brightness of the screen you're reading—especially if your eyes are sensitive to bright light—and see if your eyes feel less strained or more comfortable. A screen that is too bright can contribute to headaches, especially in people prone to migraines or other severe headaches.

43) Positioning. Remember that having a correct and comfortable distance from your eyes to the screen is critical. Discomfort or tension in your head, neck, or shoulders may be a direct result of being too near, or too far away, from your electronic reader screen. With longer periods of continuous focus, electronic readers may be a greater factor in your eye and body stress response. The positioning of any screen, however, from small phone to large television, must be thoughtfully considered. Screens are the least stressful for your body when at eye height: not too low or too high. A laptop or reader down in your lap requires your neck to bend forward; a TV screen positioned too high requires your neck to extend backwards. Such positions can cause or aggravate pain.

44) Repetitive motion. If you text or do other keyboard activities on your mobile device, pay attention to how you hold your device. Too much repetitive motion, such as constantly gripping your device one way, or using the same fingers or thumbs over and over again, can create significant pain from your hands, wrists, elbows, or shoulders up to your neck.

45) Stretches. Mini stretch breaks for your hands, arms, and eyes can help reduce the muscle tension by giving your hyper-irritated, overworked nerves a break. Your nerves are directing every movement of every muscle. Take 30-second breaks, bending your fingers and wrists in the direction opposite to your working position, and stretching your arms up overhead and out to the side and behind you. This will improve blood flow and let your nerves relax a little bit. To give your eyes a break from the intense focus, move your eye muscles to look up, down, left, and right for just 30 seconds.

46) Earbuds/Bluetooth© microphones and similar devices. If the inside of your ear feels like it's not okay, listen to your body! Try different earbuds or a different type of listening device. Even slight pressure in your ear canal can have negative effects on your muscle function. Bluetooth© devices and similar products worn outside your ear transmit EMFs directly into your body. They can cause significant muscle tension and even major pain. Try to use listening and microphone devices that do not have direct contact with your body, especially with your head. Devices anywhere on your body that transmit EMFs can impair muscle function and your goal should be to minimize those effects.

47) Headphones. Reduce the pressure of the headphones against your ears and your head as much as you can. This is especially important if you wear the device for extended periods of time. Too much pressure on the sides of your head tends to create functional problems, particularly with muscles in your shoulders and hips.

48) Constant sound and volume. Give your ears a break! Turn your listening device off periodically during the day. *Use the 60/60 rule:* Since the combination of volume and length of listening can cause hearing loss, researchers recommend applying the 60/60 rule. The rule suggests listening to a phone for 60 minutes at 60 percent of its maximum volume and then taking a break. Ears that get a rest have time to recover and are less likely to be permanently damaged. Prolonged exposure, particularly to loud noise, causes permanent damage. It is the most common cause of tinnitus, a sensation of constant "ringing" or other noise in the ear.

Research has demonstrated that even just four hours of continuous sound (at normal volumes) can have a damaging effect on the delicate sound-sensitive cells of the cochlea (the spiral-shaped organ in the inner ear) that receive the vibrations we hear as sound—whether voices, music, mechanical noise, or anything else. Long or repeated exposure to sounds at or above 85 decibels can cause hearing loss over time. (Normal conversation is around 65 decibels.) Some devices have a volume control— use it. Researchers also caution against using earbuds; they send sound straight into your ear and can boost the signal by as much as six to nine decibels. They're more likely to cause hearing damage than headphones that sit over the ear.

49) Kids and electronic devices. Children of all ages are using small-screen electronic devices, from phones to iPads® to you-name-it. Be a good role model for children, teens, and young adults. Show them *by your example* how to interact with real people, real animals, real activities, and real events in their lives. Kids are great at mimicking what the adults and older children around them are doing. If you want them to be interactive with you and their peers—and someday, with their employers—they need that real face-to-face interaction and creativity time now.

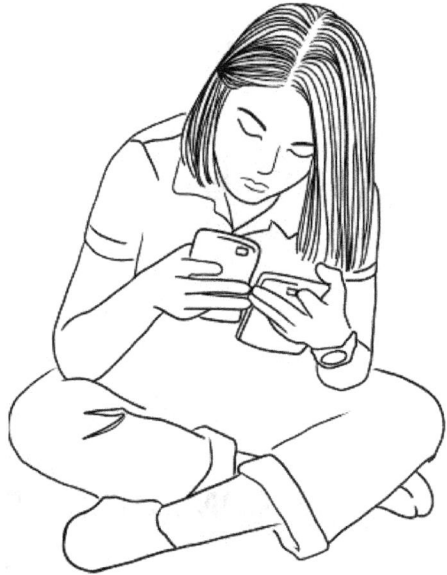

5. COMPUTERS, DESKS, & OTHER WORKSTATIONS

50) Sitting at a desk (90/90)

51) Monitor and keyboard: location

52) Mouse/trackball/ touchpad

53) Screen brightness

54) Font and image size

55) Laptop positioning

56) Desks and workstations

57) Electromagnetic fields (EMF)

58) Voice activation and dictation

59) Standing workspaces

60) Hobbies and other workplaces

61) Mats and footwear

Although small screens are becoming more and more commonplace for personal use, desktop computers, monitors, and keyboards are still the norm in many homes and workplace settings. Each device has somewhat different challenges.

50) Sitting at a desk. Have the screen directly in front of you, not off to one side. In order to determine how far away your screen should be, sit upright and reach your arm straight forward—the thumb knuckle closest to your nail should touch the screen. A posturally beneficial work position is with the keyboard height on a level with your elbows (4), elbows and knees at right angles (3), and your feet flat on the floor (5) or on a footrest. Dangling feet will tip your pelvis and put more stress on your back.

51) Monitors and keyboards: location. Adjust the height of your monitor screen so that the center of the screen is on the same level as your eyes or slightly lower. If you have to tip your head to see the screen, gravity starts pulling your head down. The muscles in your neck and back then have to tighten more to support your head position. Your neck and back muscles (1, 2) have the least amount of stress when your head is

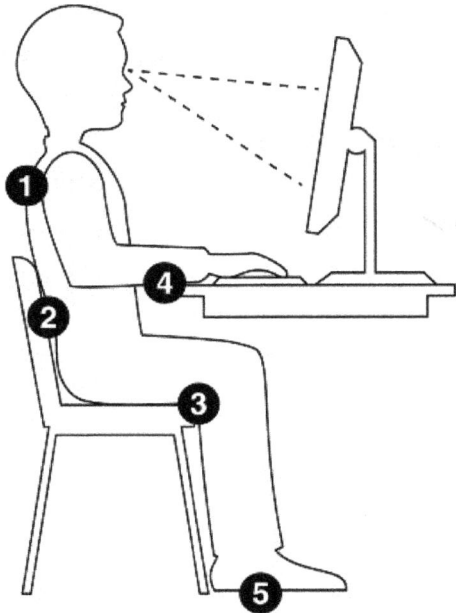

upright, with your eyes focused straight ahead. When your monitor is not properly positioned, your neck muscles will be tight all the time.

52) Mouse/trackball/touchpad. Choose the cursor control and clicking option that works best with your computer and your workstation positioning. Both elbows should be close to the side of your body. If your elbow on the mouse side is away from your body, it's much more likely to become a cause of pain. Remember, a comfortable position is less likely to create a repetitive movement disorder.

53) Screen brightness. Adjust the brightness of your screen to find a level that creates the least stress on your eyes. A screen that is too dim, or which does not have enough contrast, will create eyestrain. Too much brightness can also be stressful, especially for people with light-sensitive eyes or those who are prone to migraine headaches. (See Chapter 3 on vision, and Chapter 6 on the effects of computer and TV light on sleep patterns.)

54) Font and image size. Whether you're writing a document, working on a spreadsheet, or reading the latest news or a book on any electronic screen, adjust the size of the font and image to maximize your comfort. If your eyes are not able to comfortably process the information on the screen, your body will suffer. Your brain will shift your body in an effort to get your face and eyes into a better position. It will hunch your shoulders, tighten your neck or back muscles, thrust your chin forward—anything to try and reduce the eyestrain. If you leave any electronic screen activity with tight muscles, it might be a font-size problem.

55) Laptop positioning. The portability of laptops means your position when using one may be exacerbating your muscle tension. The preceding tips on font size are important, as are the tips on desks, chairs, and seating. An additional important tip with laptops and e-readers is to protect your body from EMF fields. When sitting with any electronic device on your legs, put a pillow, folded towel, thick magazine, or an air-circulation spacer over your legs. The longer you sit with a device on your lap, the greater the negative effects on your skin and muscles.

56) Desk/workstation. Many workstations are becoming more height-flexible, as our understanding of the downside of too much sitting has led to the development of standing or adjustable-height desks. The same basic tips apply to standard desks. Elbows need to be about the same height as your work surface and keyboard. You may need to adjust how close you are to your electronic screen as you change from one height to another: from chair, to barstool height, to standing. If you have work papers and the keyboard between you and the screen, you may find yourself pushing the monitor too far away for eye comfort.

57) Electromagnetic Fields (EMF). All electronic devices generate invisible electromagnetic fields; some devices generate more powerful fields than others. Research is continuing to show the dangers of EMF fields, although shielding is also getting better. Keep this in mind as you make decisions about where and how you use all of your electronic devices. My smartphone instruction book gives a clearly worded warning, but it's in very fine print—on page 24! I really think they don't want us to read about the potential dangers.

58) Dictation. You can reduce some of the EMFs you receive from your computer by dictating using a lightweight headset, either wired or wireless, and a software program (like Speaking Naturally® by Dragon). Unfortunately, if you're in a wireless environment, you'll be getting some EMFs anyway. The benefit is that the EMFs are not as strong or concentrated in one place on your head. You can walk to and fro while dictating with a cord about six or eight feet long. This allows for movement and even some exercise while you dictate. An additional benefit is less repetitive motion for your hands and arms and less chance of a carpal-tunnel-type problem in your wrists.

59) Standing workplaces. Speaking of standing, the majority of kitchen work at home is done standing, whether prepping food or looking up recipes on a computer. In commercial kitchens, virtually all the work is done standing. The same is true at many workbenches and lots of other jobs. Standing for extended periods of time, especially in one place, with little moving around, doesn't work well for everyone. Standing at a desk or computer workstation can be better for some people because there's less stress on the spine when standing, and the opportunity to move around is greater. However, standing workstations aren't necessarily good for everyone.

60) Hobbies and other workspaces. A computer workstation in a hobby or craft area can be at any height, but, as noted previously, be sure that your work surface and elbows are in good alignment. Also see the preceding tip on heights and be sure that your screen hasn't moved out of your visual comfort range. If you're hunching over to see your work, you probably need to raise the surface at least to where your hands and arms are more relaxed. Our eyes change over time, and lighting may need to be increased. Getting a big free-standing magnifier can be a great benefit if you need to see very fine or detailed work more clearly.

61) Mats and footwear. Any location where you do extended standing deserves a proper mat to reduce foot and leg stress. These mats are easily available online and in some stores. Good footwear that supports your arches can also make a substantial difference in how your feet and legs feel. Arch support keeps your ankles from rolling in toward each other and helps knees maintain proper alignment. Tension in the lower joints—ankles, knees, and hips—will always contribute to more tension, and often more pain, in your back and neck. This ascending pattern of tightness can also contribute to headaches and even eyestrain.

6. SLEEPING—ANYWHERE

Most of these tips apply to people of all ages. If the tip applies mostly to adults, it is so noted. Some of these tips you may never see in other information sources.

62) Mattress choices. Which is better—soft or firm? The degree of firmness that is most comfortable for you is best for you in most cases. A reasonably firm mattress will properly support your spine and body alignment. Give your body at least a week or two to adjust if you're sleeping on a mattress that's new, or new to you. Most mattresses won't last more than about eight years; less if you are (or your sleeping partner is) heavy or the mattress gets a lot of action (from adults or kids!)

63) Memory Foam®. This is currently being touted as "the best" surface for mattresses, but be aware that heat softens a memory-foam mattress. The mattress will soften in the area where your body heat is the greatest. After a few hours, it won't be as supportive as when you first laid down. Because of this softening, you may sink down into the mattress—and then changing your position during

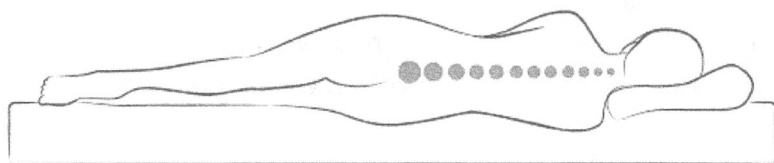

sleep may be less likely. When you spend too long in the same position, it can be less restful than moving from time to time during the night. Lack of movement can also contribute to waking with more pain.

64) Pillows. Most Americans use a pillow that is too thick. If you're sleeping lying on your back, the pillow should be just thick enough to keep your head in alignment with your spine. That means your face is parallel to the surface of the bed. If the pillow tips your chin toward your chest, it's probably too big and fluffy. If you sleep on your side, the pillow should just fill the space between your shoulder and your head (see illustration). It shouldn't tip the top of your head toward the other shoulder. Again, think good spine alignment. No one pillow filling is best, but it does help to have a filling type that you can punch into a shape that is comfortable. I'm not a fan of the chiropractic type of pillow that attempts to create a particular cervical (neck) position.

65) Magnets in bed. Please, no! Humans have lived for many thousands of years adapted to Earth's magnetic gravity field. On a living body, the polarity of a magnet (its positive or negative charge) either draws fluids to the area where it's located or drives fluids out of the area. This has definite effects on the function of the body. Under the management of a trained physician, prescribed amounts of magnetic energy can have a medical benefit, but don't be fooled by salespeople who just want to sell you magnets for profit. Something that appears to provide a benefit at the moment may actually cause dysfunction at that location or elsewhere in your body, now or later, as your body responds to the changes.

66) Crystals. I believe that the jury is still out on the benefits of crystals. The energy of crystals that occur in nature is a somewhat different matter; some people use pads embedded with crystals for their beneficial properties. I don't have enough information at this time to comment on them. Although they seem to be helpful for some people, their energetic field may not be beneficial for everyone.

67) Recliners. Recliners can be great for a short nap, but using a recliner as your primary sleep location can cause or aggravate functional problems or pain. Some of the problems with recliners are:

a. They don't allow much change of position.

b. They keep the hips in a flexed position.

c. They keep the knees flexed.

d. They generally tip the head forward.

e. The head usually rolls either left or right, toward the side that is already shorter and tighter.

These postural conditions do not help correct musculoskeletal problems. If you're not able to get to sleep on a bed or other flat surface, you should probably be seeing a health care person who can help you find out why.

68) Futons. Some futons have a flat, reasonably firm pad, such as foam rubber, and can be satisfactory for sleeping, at least for the short term. However, if the padding is irregular, tufted, or lumpy, then sleeping on it can mean an achy body the next day. Lumpy sleeping surfaces are never a good choice.

69) Sleeping on the floor. A mattress on a solid surface on the floor, or a platform bed, usually provides very firm support and can offer better sleep for some people. A thin pad that can be rolled up or folded away can likewise be perfectly adequate for kids or some adults.

70) Camping. The levelness of the surface can be critical. If the sleeping site is even slightly sloped, put your head on the higher end. Try not to have the right side of your body on the upslope and your left side on the downslope (or vice versa). That kind of sideways positioning on a slope can cause body pain the next day.

71) Light from electronic devices. Research has shown that the light from TVs, computers, e-readers, and phones, when viewed within an hour before bedtime, is likely to interfere with sleep for many individuals. This is especially true if you have difficulty falling asleep. For the last hour or two before bedtime, plan not to use electronic devices or screens. An eye mask can provide more darkness for those who are sensitive to light when sleeping.

72) Body Readiness. To bring on sleep, our body makes several adjustments. One of these is lowering the body temperature. Another is producing melatonin. Melatonin levels rise around midnight to help the mind and body go to sleep. If you have lights out by midnight, it will help your body benefit from the rise in melatonin. This can assist you in getting to sleep. Quiet music in a darkened room also helps some people get to sleep.

73) Noise. Our hearing is the last sense to turn off as we fall asleep. Noise keeps some people from getting to sleep, or it interrupts them during sleep. Try different ways to dampen auditory stimulation. If noise in the environment is outside of your control, try earplugs (inexpensive and easily portable). Some earplugs fit in the ear canal; others are soft and larger and rest in the outer part of the ear. Some people find a device that creates "white noise" helpful. White noise is like gentle rain, a distant waterfall, etc., and even when the volume is very low, the sound wavelength masks annoying sounds. A small white noise device, a CD, or an app on a cell phone can provide this kind of soothing sound.

7. WHAT YOU WEAR—ANYWHERE

74) Support hose/stockings

75) Socks

76) Jeans

77) Special-use pants

78) Helmets and other protective head gear

79) Other hats and caps

80) Hairstyles? Yes, hairstyles

81) Jewelry

82) Magnetized jewelry

83) Sensitivity to touch

84) Skin sensitivity

85) Back braces & joint braces

It may seem unlikely, but some jeans, other clothes, jewelry, hats, and hair accessories can create discomfort! (For socks—see Shoes, Tip #12.)

74) Support hose. Support hose, compression hose, and support nylons are needed or helpful for some health conditions that affect the feet or legs. **Follow the recommendations of your health care provider!** My clinical experience seems to indicate that if the size is correct, support hose do not seem to affect muscle function. However, if your foot or leg size changes, you may require a different size.

75) Socks. If your socks encircle the arch of your foot with reinforced elastic bands, those bands interfere with nerve signals to your brain about the position of your foot. This is also true of low-cut socks that have an elastic band at the top of the sock, which encircles and ends on your ankle bones. These ankle elastics may also cause problems. Elastic bands around either the arch of the foot or around the ankle affect muscle function all the way up your spine and neck.

TIP: If you like low-cut socks, find low-cut athletic socks that end *below* your ankle bones— and be sure they do *not* have reinforced elastic bands around the arches.

76) Jeans. Americans (and many others) love jeans. They can be great, and skinny stretch jeans are usually okay.

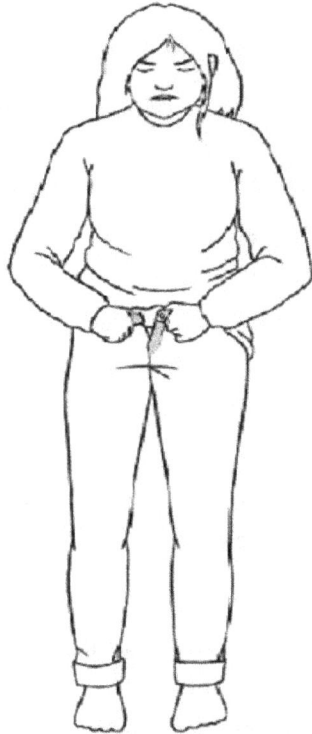

Problems can occur when the not-so-stretchy jeans become too tight. (*"The dryer shrank them!"*) The strong weave of the fabric and double-heavy seams can result in compression of your hips and sacroiliac joints (at the end of your spine). That compression affects the function of your muscles so they can't work up to par. The result can be hip pain, back pain, or even headaches. Yes, really. If you have to suck in your tummy to button or zip your jeans, they're probably compressing your pelvic joints and having a bad effect on your nerves and muscles. In order to be more comfortable and to help your body function better, wear jeans that aren't so tight.

77) Special-use pants. These are used for many sports, horseback riding, etc. Some clothing in this group has a band that goes under the arch of your foot to keep the pants leg from creeping upward. These under-the-arch straps can increase tension in the bottom of the feet and back of the legs, and all the way up the spine to your head. This tension can cause or aggravate pain in any of these areas. Tightness in the back of your body also causes your flexor muscles (on the front of your body) to work less effectively. Try to minimize use of under-the-arch bands and adjust them to be less tight when such clothing is essential.

78) Helmets and other protective headgear. First, the headbands or helmets medically recommended for some infants and very young children are fine. They're carefully custom-designed and regularly monitored. They're helpful, not harmful, and are very important to improving a child's growth and development. Protective helmets for many sports, including all kinds of cycle riding, are also very important, as they help protect the brain and reduce traumatic injury. They should be individually selected, then adjusted to provide the best fit and protection. You only have one brain. Do everything possible to protect it.

79) Other hats and caps. If the band on a hat, such as a baseball cap, is too tight, it can cause headaches. The tight band can also impair and compromise muscle function in other parts of your body, causing muscles to fatigue more quickly. This fix is easy. Loosen the adjustable band on your cap or buy a larger size if you need to. You'll be more comfortable during your golf game or other sport, and your scores may even improve!

80) Hairstyles? Yes, hairstyles. Ponytails pulled tight, and elastic-type hairbands, are the most likely styles to cause headaches or muscle aches, but the plastic or metal hairbands that are shaped like an arch often put pressure (above or behind your ears) on the temporal bones. This pressure can cause pain in your hips and shoulders or cause headaches. Cornrows and other tight braids usually pull the scalp tight, but since each braid typically pulls from a relatively small area, it seems that braided hairstyles do not usually create musculoskeletal problems. Hairstyles that include substantial hair additions, like dreadlocks, may put more stress on the scalp if they're heavy, and may therefore cause tension or pain in your head or neck. Give your hairstyle some thought if you have pain in your head, neck, or shoulders. Try a less stressful hairstyle for a week or two and see if your symptoms are less, or in different parts of your body.

81) Jewelry. Jewelry that causes a problem for your body can be tight, magnetized, or simply irritating. Wristwatches and bracelets that are tight enough to leave a red imprint on your arm can cause dysfunction or pain at the fingers, wrist, or elbow. If they're very tight, the tightness can even affect shoulder muscles. If ordinary necklaces feel irritating, the reason may be hyper-irritated nerves, which are probably the same nerves causing your neck and shoulder muscles to be very tight and painful. Therapy that reduces your neck and shoulder tension may also let you be more comfortable wearing some necklaces.

82) Magnetized jewelry. Any jewelry that is magnetized will cause tension in some muscles and reduce the energy available to other (opposing) muscles. Pain can result, especially if this jewelry is worn frequently. Our bodies have lived with Earth's magnetic gravitational field for thousands of years and are adapted to its magnetic field. There are valid medical uses for magnets, but any magnets on your body should only be those prescribed and monitored by a physician trained in their use, for a very specific reason and a specific time.

83) Sensitivity to touch (or sound). (May be called "sensory defensiveness.") If children (or adults) are unusually sensitive to tags in clothing, the feel of fabrics, or the texture of certain foods, then the body's neurological system may be hypersensitive to touch (tactile sensitivity) or not well integrated neurologically. Reducing overall stress in the body may help. This includes reducing physical and emotional stress, as well as foods that may be causing inflammation—an internal stress that we often do not recognize unless it appears as a rash. Sensory integration therapy is a treatment that can be very effective in reducing such sensitivity. It tends to improve both comfort and behavior, especially in children, but it is also helpful for adults with sensory defensiveness. Sensory integration therapy is provided by some occupational therapists, and also by other specially trained health care providers.

84) Skin sensitivity. Irritation can be caused by laundry detergents, fabric softeners, body soaps, lotions, or chemically treated garments. Rashes can also be caused by your body's reaction to certain foods, or to chemicals in your home, neighborhood, or workplace. See if changing some of those aspects of your "personal environment" reduces your skin problems. It is also a good idea to seek out the most natural products available. Sometimes skin problems indicate a deeper health care issue; if your symptoms persist more than a couple of weeks, see a health care provider, such as a dermatologist (a specialist in skin disorders).

85) Back braces and joint braces. Sometimes a back brace for heavy work, or a knee or elbow brace for sports activities, is a necessity. However, such devices can also become a crutch that simply suppresses your awareness of symptoms that should be receiving some kind of physical therapy or medical attention. Masking pain can allow a problem to become worse if you continue to overstress or overwork the joint and associated muscles. If symptoms persist more than a week or two, see a local health care provider.

8. THE STUFF YOU CARRY AROUND

86) Wallets, phones, and more
87) Purses
88) Bookbags and backpacks
89) Fanny packs
90) Briefcases
91) Pull-behind suitcases
92) Suitcases—four-wheeled spinners
93) Carrying infants
94) Carrying toddlers

95) Toolboxes
96) Boxes
97) Lifting

We often give very little thought to the various kinds of stuff that we tote around, sometimes every day. Wallets, purses, briefcases, backpacks—the list gets long. It can pay to give some consideration to these activities; there are ways to make carrying things easier and much more comfortable for your body.

86) Wallets, phones, and more. You'll probably end up sitting on anything you carry in your hip pocket, causing your pelvis to tilt and rotate every time you sit down. Just. Stop. Now! Hip-pocket items are almost a guarantee for long-term posture and pain problems. (This common bad habit keeps many chiropractors busy; the really good ones remind you frequently to keep those hip pockets empty.) Sciatic nerve pain in the buttocks, hips, or legs is one of the most frequent symptoms that your pelvis is tipped. If one hip is higher than the other for months, pain is a common result—maybe now, maybe later. Carry your stuff somewhere else and spend less on doctors and therapy in the future. Pad your wallet, not theirs.

87) Purses. Many purses are okay if they're carried in your hand or in a diagonal strap across your body. Carrying any bag or tote on one shoulder creates a twist in your body and causes muscle imbalance. Frequent or long-term carrying like this is very likely to result in pain somewhere in your body. The area of pain may vary depending on your body's other problems. The easy solution is to use purses and bags that have a long enough strap to go across to your opposite shoulder and hang on the diagonal, or a short handle that you carry in your hand.

88) Bookbags and backpacks. Bookbag purses, or their larger cousins, backpacks, are designed to be carried on your back with the weight equally distributed between both shoulders. A healthy child, teen, or adult should be able to carry up to about one third of their body weight on their back (e.g., 20 pounds of books for a 60-pound kid).

Complaints about bookbags that are too heavy are likely to be a kid just whining, or may be the result of carrying that bookbag on one shoulder. Or maybe they just need more physical exercise that will develop their core strength.

89) Fanny packs. Fanny packs are worn in the front or on the center back, which is fine. If they're more than eight ounces and are worn regularly on one hip or the other, they can cause muscular stress.

90) Briefcases. Briefcases that are carried only a short distance and not too many times a day should not usually cause physical discomfort. However, carrying one often on the same side, especially for long walks through buildings

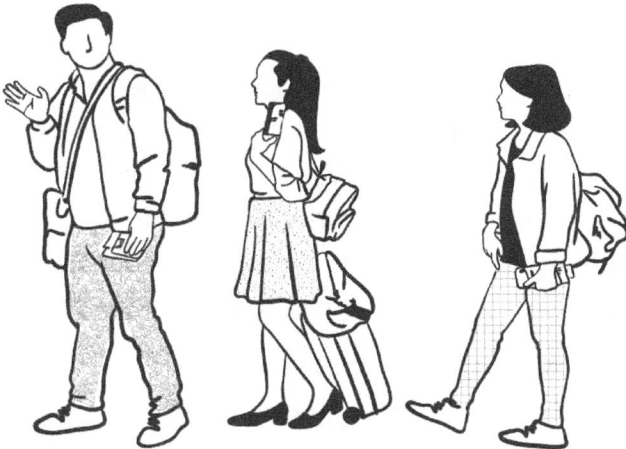

or airports, twists the spine and creates muscle imbalances that may develop into pain patterns sooner or later. If you're toting a briefcase frequently, consider getting one with wheels. It will be money well spent.

91) Pull-behind suitcases. Suitcases that are pulled behind are very likely to cause the body to twist. If you drag the suitcase further behind you, the pains or problems can be worse. Usually one shoulder or arm is doing all the work in that position. Keeping the arm that is pulling close to your hip tends to minimize problems; so will switching sides if you have a long walk. If you have two suitcases, pulling one behind you in each hand is better but is still not good and is certainly very stressful. If you travel often, consider other kinds of suitcases.

92) Suitcases—four-wheeled spinners. Suitcases with four wheels make it easy to keep your arm close to your side and are a far better choice than pulling a suitcase behind you. Your arm is still somewhat out to your side, but the position is less stressful. If done for a long time, or frequently, this position can cause a problem in the middle deltoid muscle of your upper arm, or pain in the side of your hip. It's still a better choice than pulling a suitcase behind you. You can work to strengthen the opposing muscles, which pull your elbows in close to your ribs.

93) Carrying infants. Babies love to be carried on your body, and carrying them centered in front or centered in back is best for a parent, and, in many ways, is also better for the baby. Carrying an infant on one side, on your hip, creates a body position that is not good posture and can contribute to muscle or joint pain. Do whatever you can to avoid side-carrying an infant on a frequent basis or on a long outing. Infant car seats—which work wonderfully well in a car—are very difficult on an adult's body when carried outside the car. Do this only for a very short distance, and switch the side you are carrying on frequently, especially if your arm or body starts to ache.

94) Carrying toddlers. Carrying a toddler on one hip for any more than a very short distance is a sure recipe for muscle pain and postural distortion. This is doubly true if it's an older child. When a youngster who is still growing is carrying a younger child, or even other loads on one side, it's more likely to create nerve and muscle changes that may last for many years. If you're in a situation where you expect to carry a toddler frequently, use a backpack, stroller, or other system that's designed for carrying a toddler. That expense will be offset in the money you will save on doctors or pain management later.

95) Toolboxes. Carrying a toolbox on a jobsite is sometimes an unavoidable situation. It's important to consider how this stress may be affecting your ability to do the job that the tools require. Try to find a workaround that will help you to avoid carrying a toolbox any more than is absolutely essential.

96) Boxes. We all encounter the need to carry boxes sometimes, whether we're packing and moving, or just moving objects from one area to another. How you carry those boxes can make a big difference in whether or not you have pain or an injury as a result. The best choice is to have some kind of wheeled device to help you transport those boxes from point A to point B, but this is obviously not always an option.

Ideally, when you're picking up a box, it should be close to waist height. If that's not an option, then your feet should be *pointing at the box* when you pick it up. Bend your knees and lift from a squatting position, using your leg muscles to do the heavy lifting, not your spine and back muscles. Bring the box to waist height, holding it close to your body. Now, *after* you are standing upright, you can safely turn around to set the box down, or walk with it.

Special Tip

If you're moving multiple boxes, take a break now and then. Sit down and do this little exercise: Tighten your tummy muscles (your abdominals) and lean forward. Bring your arms underneath your knees and hug your chest down to your knees. Let your head hang down between your knees for 5 to 15 seconds, then slowly sit up. You can repeat this little stretch two or three times. It helps your back muscles relax, even if you just do it for a few minutes before you resume your box-carrying task. Your back muscles will thank you. If you do have sore muscles afterward, and the symptoms don't go away in two or three days, you should see a medical professional to be sure you haven't created (or aggravated) a joint or muscle problem.

---

97) Lifting. Learning how to lift properly and use your joints correctly in any activity is always a good idea. Strengthening the muscles in your legs and trunk may help your joints work more effectively and enable you to work more safely. These are good long-term strategies and may provide relief in some cases. However, any joint under repetitive stress, whether at work or during recreational activities, needs medical attention if dysfunction or pain persists. Joint replacements are just not as good as your original parts. Take care of your joints. They're very important moving parts of the vehicle you call your body!

9. LEISURE ACTIVITIES

98) Drinking water

99) Recreational activities and pain

100) Stretching

101) Sports with even, bilateral movement

102) Sports with uneven movements

103) Kids and sports

104) Falls and other traumas

105) Blows to the head; concussions

106) Yoga and tai chi

107) Social dancing

108) Gardening

109) Mountain biking, rock climbing, and extreme sports

Some of us are capable of and inclined toward active movement—whether competitively, for pleasure, for the socializing benefits, or just to stay healthier and in better shape. This leisure list is very broad; it includes gardening, and even video game binges (lots of fast muscle action there for thumbs and wrists). We may not consider some of the less-than-ideal aspects of our favorite recreation when we're out just having fun. If you or your loved ones (of any age) engage in any active leisure pursuits, here are some tips.

98) Drinking water. When you're being physically active, plain water is often not enough. Staying adequately hydrated during any physical activity is essential. When you perspire, your body loses salt and other minerals in that sweat. Your body needs those minerals; it must have them for nerves to communicate with other nerves and your muscles. If you drink too much water and don't replace the lost electrolytes (minerals), your nerves can't fire properly. You'll tire more quickly because your muscles aren't firing like they should. The nerves in your brain also slow down. If you lose too many electrolytes, your brain will eventually power down, and you will pass out. This is known as heatstroke. There are many beverage choices for replenishing your electrolytes. If you're working up a sweat doing anything, find a good way to replace those lost electrolytes while your brain is still talking to you.

99) Recreational activities and pain. Recreation can be almost anything we consider fun—from video games to mountain climbing and all manner of things in between. You can't enjoy your favorite recreational activities, however, if you have tight muscles telling you that they need a break. For a quick break, move your muscles in the opposite direction. If you've been reaching forward, reach back! If you've been reaching down, reach up! Stretch them out, gently but firmly. Pain in your body is the way muscles and joints say that you have overworked or injured them. Stop what you are doing. Let your body, muscles, and joints relax and recover. Pain is your body's cry for help. Listen! If the pain is serious, get a professional opinion and appropriate help before you cause long-term damage. Then choose activities and duration accordingly, so you can have fun for many years to come.

100)   Stretching. Stretching is probably the least expensive and best thing that you can do to help your body remain mobile and active throughout your life. A general rule is light stretching before a physical activity, followed by more stretching after your activity. The stretching before gets more blood flowing to your muscles and warms them up for action. Afterward, stretching can help tight muscles relax and recover. On a computer, in the kitchen, outside on a ladder, or on the sports field—wherever you are working or playing, give your muscles that much-needed stretching. If you're doing workouts in a gym, a general rule of thumb is 20 minutes of stretching for each hour of workout.

101)   Sports that have even, bilateral movement. Sports with bilateral movement are better for developing well-balanced muscles because muscle movement is relatively equal on both your right side and your left side. Some sports that fit this category are bicycling, swimming, walking, running, snow skiing, and kayaking. You may still need to consider the needs of your upper body versus your lower body, but your nervous system likes the equality of left, right, left, right rhythm. Basketball is an example of an in-between sport. The running is bilateral, but most people do more dribbling and basket-shooting with their dominant hand, so movements are less even.

102)   Sports   with   uneven   movements.   From shuffleboard and pickle ball to ping-pong, tennis, bowling, and golf, there are many sports with uneven muscle movements. Baseball and softball are also prime examples. When you use your muscles repetitively in unbalanced ways, patterns of tight muscles and uneven muscle development will typically create pain over time (like "tennis elbow"). Make an effort to develop muscles on the opposite side to extend your enjoyment of favorite activities.

103)   Kids and sports. Individual and team activities— from the brain workout of chess to bike races, basketball, martial arts, and many other sports—can help a child develop physical, mental, social, and emotional skills. These are all good reasons to encourage the children in your life to participate in one or more sports that fit each child's needs and talents. It helps to be aware that in children, just as in adults, sensitivity to pain varies greatly from one person to another. We now know that one's genes can be a factor in pain sensitivity. A person who is highly sensitive to pain will be less likely to enjoy rough-and-tumble sports; he or she will be more likely to choose activities that are less physically demanding or which have less physical contact with others.

Repetition of specific movements is required to develop physical skills, especially in sports. During childhood and through the teen years, muscles are growing to keep up with growing bones, as are the nerves that control those muscles. It is my professional clinical experience that children who engage in intensive repetitive practice—especially in a single sport for months on end—may develop repetitive motion disorders at a relatively early age, even before adulthood. Encouraging a variety of activities during the year and different roles within a single sport are both ways to help a young person develop more balanced function in his or her nerves, muscles, and postural/skeletal systems.

104)   Falls and other traumas. Some sports have a much greater likelihood of falls, body blows, and other traumas. Even though children typically bounce back quickly from a fall, or appear to recover easily from an impact that causes some obvious injury, the nerves and muscles are recording these traumas. And as I like to tell my patients, the body is like an elephant—it never forgets. Sprains, breaks, and other nerve/muscle dysfunctions that happen in childhood can set the stage for other physical problems to surface many years later. At any age, the complaints of a young person should be taken seriously when they report lingering pain from an impact, sore joints/muscles, or discomfort that is frequent or chronic. Adults should seek care a day or two after any fall or trauma. The body doesn't lie (although sometimes you may have a hard time understanding what it's trying to tell you).

TIP: Continuing to play when you have pain is just asking for trouble (regardless of your age). When nerves and muscles aren't functioning properly, other muscles and joints are also out of balance as they try to pick up the slack. Falls and other injuries are more likely because the workload is not being shared equally. Don't ignore pain, and don't just cover it up. That's like putting a Band-Aid across your motor vehicle's overheating symbol. Your recognition of the problem is suppressed, but it can be getting worse while you pretend it's not important. Not a good idea in either case.

105)   Blows to the head; concussions. We know a lot more about concussions now than we did a few years ago. Research has shown that falls and blows to the head that seem minor are still contributing to a pattern of brain injury. The more repetitions, the greater the damage. If you have any question about having received a concussion, see a health care provider promptly. Those repeated incidents are causing changes that can lead to long-term brain dysfunction, including dementia and Alzheimer's disease.

Children and teens are most at risk because their brains are still developing many nerve connections. Attention deficit disorder (ADD) and attention deficit/ hyperactivity disorder (ADHD) have been linked to head trauma. A concussion at any age can cause headaches or brain fog and interrupt cognitive processing—that precious ability to focus on a task, think about problems, learn new material, and make good decisions. A concussion can also affect emotional processing, so, for example, a person who has suffered a concussion may be more short-tempered or quick to laugh or cry. These behavioral changes may be seen in children, teens, and adults. Protect your brain. Your success in learning new skills, career activities, and relationships, as well as your long-term health, are all much better with an undamaged brain!

TIP: Avoid activities that are likely to result in blows to your head. Always buckle your seatbelt. Don't put a vehicle in gear until everyone is buckled in. Always wear the appropriate protective helmet for your activities. Be aware of the potentially dangerous consequences of head trauma from any source, including slip-and-fall accidents, motor vehicle accidents, and fights. A bruise inside the head can cause internal bleeding, headaches, a stroke, and even death. Take blows to the head and concussions seriously! Don't take chances; if your head takes a hard blow, see a medical doctor and *get your head examined!*

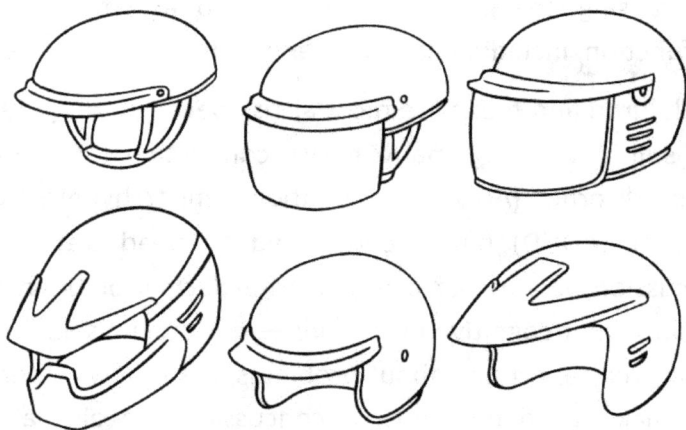

106) **Yoga and tai chi.** Yoga and tai chi have become popular for very good reasons. They're low impact, so generally safe for knees and hips, and they help maintain and improve muscle function and coordination. Regular practice also improves joint range of motion, balance, and strength. Research into the benefits of tai chi has shown improvement in bone density in seniors in just six months of three-times-a-week practice. These activities promote mental focus and emotional tranquility and are also suitable for any age group. No special clothing or equipment is required, and the exercises can be done inside or outside, making them an excellent year-round choice for individual or group exercise that is safe and beneficial. Participate at your own pace; your skills will develop over time.

107) **Social dancing.** There are many different kinds of dance, and it provides good exercise at any age. Dancing offers many benefits in the context of social interaction, and the skill and physical difficulty level can vary widely, even at one social dancing location or event. The level of cardio and aerobic activity also varies greatly, depending on the type of dance and the intensity of your involvement. The advantages include (usually) a non-competitive environment where both beginners and the more experienced can enjoy each other's company, and each person can participate at a level that his or her joint mobility and energy permits. The tip here is to find the kind of dancing that you like and go for the enjoyment of socializing, music, and movement, regardless of your skills.

The benefits for your body can be significant with regular participation.

108)   Gardening. This leisure activity can be pursued at almost any level; land ownership is not required! Although most gardening is done outside, indoor plants and terrariums also count! The pleasure of working with living plants can be calming and healing, in and of itself. Gardening has many benefits, including being outdoors, a variety of movements, exercise, and visible results. And if you so choose, your results can be edible—from herbs to vegetables. Gardening can be done at your own pace and on a scale of your choice, whether hydroponic gardening, on a small balcony with potted plants, in a big yard, or in a community garden where space, tools, and tasks are shared according to interests and abilities. Gauge your physical abilities and skills so you don't overdo things, especially if you're working alone outdoors. Be particularly careful on ladders. And finally, especially in the warmer months, be sure to stay hydrated.

109)   Mountain biking, rock climbing, and extreme sports. These sports (and similar ones) are for strong, fit, and hardy individuals. If you haven't been working out, toning and strengthening your muscles, and developing good cardiac conditioning and lung capacity, do yourself and others a favor: pass on these activities. Strenuous activities like these require stamina that isn't acquired in just a couple of weeks. If you are not truly ready for the level of exertion that is required, you put yourself and maybe others at risk.

If there's an activity that you really want to do, then set your goal and create a readiness schedule. Work your way up to those higher performance levels. Dedicate yourself to the hours and months that are required to do these activities safely. Then you can enjoy the adventure!

10. WHAT'S THAT I SMELL?

Odors surround us, both manmade and natural. Although many people are not aware of negative effects, some odors may be affecting your health in ways you don't suspect. Read this chapter carefully if you or anyone you care about has sinus or respiratory problems. Some people are easily affected by many odors. Being aware of the influence of odors may help your health or could help you be more considerate of your partner, your friends, your coworkers, or people near you at any group event.

110) **Personal fragrances.** Odors affect your nervous system and sinus cavities. The air spaces in your nose, face, and forehead can become uncomfortably swollen or infected when you have a cold or when your olfactory (smelling) nerves are irritated. Your external environment (any place outside of your body) can be a major source of irritation, although some people have sinus irritations in response to foods or beverages that their body cannot process effectively. If you have sinus or respiratory problems, consult appropriate health care providers, then consider the other tips in this chapter as information that may provide additional relief.

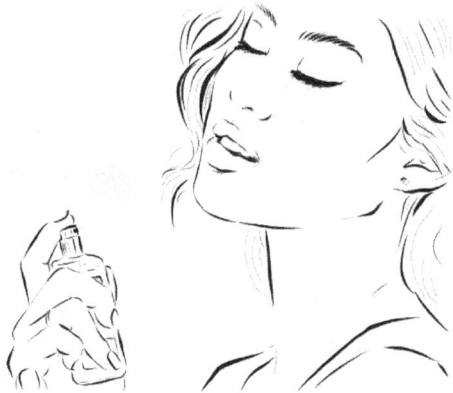

Too much scent is disrespectful. Assuming your nose is working just fine, realize that although you love a certain personal fragrance, other people may not. Even brief exposures to some aromas may cause another person to have a sudden headache or sinus irritation. If your personal fragrance is evident from more than two feet away, you are being disrespectful of other peoples' airspace. Be considerate.

111) **Odor awareness.** (Lack of awareness is sometimes referred to as "nose blind.") For most people, sensitivity to aromas declines with repeated exposure to the same odor or fragrance. Sensitivity to odors also tends to decline for many people in their senior years.

TIP: If you're over 60, be sure you're not using too much cologne or aftershave. Ask a much younger person if you're overdoing your personal fragrances. If your nose is offended by another person's use of fragrance (especially if they're older), understand that they may not be aware of how strong it is. If the situation is appropriate, try to gently educate them without being judgmental.

112) **Air pollution.** In urban environments, this is often unavoidable. The carbon monoxide pollution generated by gas and diesel-burning vehicles like cars, buses, and trucks is a headache or sinus trigger for some people. If you're one of these folks, try to limit your exposure or reduce your reaction to the exposure. Your reaction to some urban pollutants such as factory smoke, particles of soot, etc., may be reduced somewhat by use of a mask over your nose and mouth if the pollution is heavy and you can't avoid it.

113) Public and indoor air spaces. These include trains, buses, and buildings. If your exposure is relatively brief or infrequent, travel prepared with a mask, if need be, or with another product that helps you cope. Consider keeping an antihistamine (or other product) handy to help reduce your reaction to offensive or dangerous odors. If it is your workplace that has offensive odors, discuss odor issues with an appropriate supervisor or the human resources department. You have the right to air that isn't offensive or a health challenge to you.

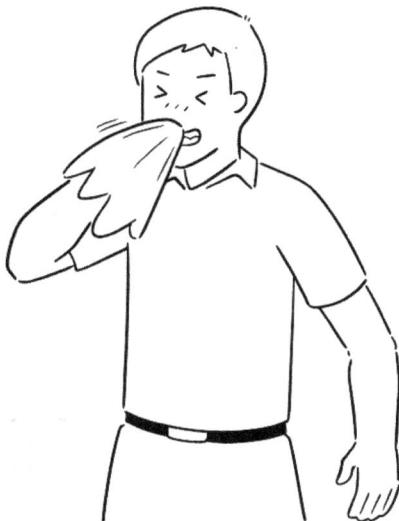

114) Places that you go. This includes stores, restaurants, concerts, churches, hotels, etc. If you can "vote with your feet and your dollars," make it a point to patronize stores and hotels that strive to minimize odors and fragrances. Let a decision-maker at the smelly location know why you're taking your business elsewhere. In churches, restaurants, and other gathering spaces or concert venues, ask to be seated (or reseated) away from a heavy scent that is creating a problem for you. You don't need to apologize; you haven't done anything wrong. It's the person (or organizational maintenance issue) that has created a problem for other patrons.

115)   Home furnishings. Upholstered furniture, many carpets, and some drapes can "outgas" from the fabrics, fibers, glues, or stuffing used in the product. Hard floorings, cabinets, and non-upholstered furniture can also outgas from the chemicals used in their construction and finishes. Any of these outgassing products can create headaches, sinus congestion, respiratory problems, or even other health problems, such as neurological symptoms or a rash. Such reactions can be a bigger problem for young children, seniors, people with other health conditions, or someone who spends many hours in that environment every day.

TIPS:

    a. Whenever possible, buy home furnishings that are months or years post-production, maybe from a showroom display, or a gently pre-owned item that can be thoroughly cleaned.

    b. If moving into a space with anything new—from paint and wall treatments to floor coverings, or anything in between—open doors and windows as often as possible, for as long as possible, to help rid the air of toxic fumes (even if you can't smell them, they're often present for weeks or months).

    c. Certain varieties of living plants are attractive houseplants (golden pothos, for example) and actually draw some undesirable chemicals out of the air. Plants also release oxygen and are nature's own air-fresheners—with no undesirable side effects.

116)   Aromatherapy. This also includes other fragrance therapy treatments. Sometimes fragrances are offered in spas and massage therapy settings. If you don't tolerate a wide variety of fragrances comfortably, be a bit cautious, and ask upfront if fragrances are used in the facility. The source of the fragrance may not matter at all. Even high-quality, "natural" essential oils can create a negative reaction in some individuals.

TIP: Be aware that a fragrance previously used in that space will often still be present, at least in trace amounts, even if you have requested no fragrance or a different fragrance.

117)   Household   fragrances/scented   products. Although intended to enhance a home's environment, artificial fragrances can create unsuspected problems. If anyone in the household has headaches, sinus issues, or respiratory problems, try eliminating all scented household products for a month or so. It may reveal that some products are irritants. This includes all plug-in products, fragrant oils with diffusing sticks, scented candles, scented cleaning products (including laundry detergents, fabric softeners, and static-free products for your dryer), and dusting and polishing products. The same is true of scented products for vacuum cleaners. Skip using them. Save money and your health! It's a win-win!

118) Spills and pets and odors. Clean up any liquid spills on carpets promptly to avoid the development of odors and mold or mildew; once started, mold can grow (unseen and unnoticed) into a big and expensive-to-remove problem. If you have pets that use indoor litter pads or boxes, avoid products that are artificially fragranced. A better choice is a product that absorbs and neutralizes the odors by natural chemical reactions. Empty and clean your pets' litter box often as the odors can be not only unpleasant but actually very unhealthy to breathe. After pet accidents, use a pet odor-neutralizer to cancel the odor, not a fragrance to just perfume the air.

119) Paint and other interior finishes. Many of these products are now available in what are called "low VOC" formulas, meaning they are low in volatile organic compounds. (Volatile organic compounds—VOCs—are organic chemicals that are emitted as gases from certain solids or liquids at ordinary room temperature. They are both natural and man-made, and many are hazardous to human health.) Use the low-odor alternatives whenever possible; they're a safer and healthier choice. Wood-staining products and paint-stripping products often have very heavy and toxic VOC odors. Activities involving these products should be done outside whenever possible, or if done indoors, they should be used when residents can be away, and with a lot of ventilation. The chemical odors of these products can cause sinus, throat, and respiratory problems when these products are used in inhabited buildings, and the odors can persist indoors for many days after their application.

120)   Cars, trucks, and motor homes. The same tips that apply to your home also apply to the interior spaces of your vehicles (See #6 on outgassing and #8 and #9 on fragrances). Maybe more so, because you can't just go to another room. It's better to get rid of fragrance devices that may dangle from your rearview mirror and not use fragranced cleaning products or polishes on the interior of your vehicles. (If you have a brand-new vehicle, use every possible opportunity to have the windows open and let the outgassing clear.) Remove open food and drink containers so they don't have a chance to develop mold. Put small open boxes of baking soda under the seats in your truck or car to help absorb unwanted odors.

121)   Outdoors. Usually, natural environments with abundant trees and plants, or wide-open spaces like deserts with moving fresh air, are naturally self-cleaning spaces where the air is fresher and less polluted. Saltwater shores and deep forests also have very cleansing air. Areas that have blossoming plants with heavy fragrances (like magnolias, gardenias, lilacs, etc.) can be a bit much for people who are fragrance sensitive, even though they're beautiful to others. Swampy and very humid areas may have high mold or mildew counts that can also cause sinus headaches and other health problems for sensitive individuals. Know your body's triggers and seek outdoor spaces where you can enjoy the benefits of our natural world without adverse body reactions.

11. THE ENERGY AROUND US

(Electronics, magnetic items, vibration, and other energy influences)

122) Magnetic cards

123) Wearable magnets

124) Magnets in your environment

125) Wearable electronic devices

126) Smart watches

127) Wireless networks, anywhere

128) Earth's negative ion field

129) 60 Hz sensitivity

130) Vibration

131) Crystals

132) Medical electronic implants

133) Other subtle energies

The presence of 60 Hz electric fields (the transmitting frequency of electrical wires and appliances throughout our homes and communities in the USA) began over 100 years ago with the inventions of Thomas Edison and Alexander Graham Bell when they brought us electric lights and the earliest telephones, respectively. Now the electromagnetic fields (EMF) of our computers and countless wireless devices affect us almost everywhere we go. This chapter discusses ways to minimize the negative effects of energy fields that we can measure, especially those that are much stronger, like high voltage electrical transmission lines, or those that we spend many hours very close to, like our cell phones and smartwatches, which may be harmful, especially when exposure exists for an extended period or the energy field is strong.

122) **Magnetic cards.** All life on our planet exists in Earth's magnetic field. Over thousands of years, our bodies have developed to function in this particular magnetic field. Elaborate scientific studies have been done on astronauts to document the way their bodies change in the absence of Earth's magnetic field; the changes in their body functions are not beneficial.

It seems very surprising, but even the amount of magnetism in the magnetic strip on a credit card (or any other membership or access card) can affect muscle function when it's in close contact with your body! If your magnetic cards are in your wallet, or in a purse or backpack, you have enough separation. However, if you carry a card with a magnetic strip in your pocket for easy access, slip it into one of the RFID sleeves that are cheap and readily available. Those sleeves protect your body, and also prevent dishonest people from scanning your card information with special remote devices (which can be some distance from you).

123) Wearable magnets. Medical science has identified ways to use certain levels of positive or negative magnetic fields for specific benefits. Such uses are prescribed in specific ways and monitored for placement, the polarity of the magnetic field, and the length of time they're used. These kinds of medical uses have been researched, and the benefits for bone and soft tissue healing have been documented.

On the other hand, magnets sold commercially as bracelets, necklaces, rings, etc., provide unknown levels of magnetic strength and are not designed specifically for you. Commercial "jewelry" magnets can have harmful consequences, especially if worn or used frequently. Spend your money more wisely! Seek out a licensed health care provider to care for joint and muscle aches or other physical symptoms.

124) **Magnets in your environment.** Generally speaking, avoid bed pads or chair pads with embedded magnets. The same goes for magnets embedded in a belt or inserted in shoes. Having a magnetic personality can be very desirable, but you won't get it by wearing magnets!

125) **Wearable electronic listening devices.** Bluetooth® and other brands of cellular communication devices, which are designed to be worn in or on your ears, on your head, or hanging around your neck, are putting the EMF frequencies in very close proximity to your brain. And you must know that your brain is a very finely tuned bioelectrical computer that is running 24/7. The soft tissues of your scalp, your temporalis jaw muscles, and your neck muscles are all directly affected by devices at your ear so that your nerves, muscles, and organs are put under stress and can't function the way they're supposed to. In short, electrical devices worn on or around your head can be creating detrimental effects on your health, and the extent of dysfunction they're likely to cause in the body is not well understood. Minimize your use of them to reduce stress on your body.

126) Fitness trackers, smartwatches, and other wearable microcomputers. These devices may offer great convenience, but it appears that wearing them may come with a price that goes above and beyond the dollars you paid for them. The level and amount of micro-current and EMFs they produce is sure to be different from one device and brand to another, and people do have different tolerances, but be aware that they can affect muscles and other body functions. Erring on the side of safety—if any of these devices has GPS tracking (and most of them do), other individuals or organizations may be able to track all of your movements whenever the GPS is active. Maybe you want someone to know where you are … but maybe not just anybody.

127) **A wireless network.** In your home or workplace, a wireless network saturates your environment with EMF waves. As of this writing, we do not yet know what the long-term effects may be of such exposure. Wireless networks are energy fields that our bodies are not acclimated to. More good research is needed. Make an effort to learn about new scientific findings on the effects of EMF waves on the human body as they become available. Try to minimize the time you spend in wireless network fields, especially if you have pain or other health challenges.

128) **Earth's negative ion field.** Get "grounded." In its most simple form, you can "plug in" to Mother Earth by direct contact of skin on the ground—walking barefoot on a path, lying in damp grass, or on the sand at a beach. Even better is having your feet or body in any natural body of water. Humans have evolved in Earth's electromagnetic field; Earth's electrical field has a powerful beneficial influence on the physiological processes of our bodies 24/7. It affects the function of individual cells, blood pressure, inflammation, and much more. My personal favorite for a good, thorough, and very readable book on this topic is *Earthing* (2014) by Ober, Sinatra, and Zucker. Chapter 8 has many references to recent research. Direct contact with the Earth allows the overly <u>positive</u> electrical charge of your body to become more balanced by taking up Earth's naturally <u>negative</u> charge. Recent studies indicate that being physically "grounded" with the Earth can be not only calming, but it can also demonstrate measurable benefits on physical healing.

Recognizing that this type of direct natural grounding contact is not practical for everyone, grounding (also called "earthing") pads can provide a similar benefit. These specially designed mats or metal plates are for use indoors. They connect your body with the Earth's natural electrical field using only the grounding opening of a modern three-prong electrical outlet. Being physically connected to Earth's natural energy field of negative ions appears to offer a healing power that too few of us use anymore.

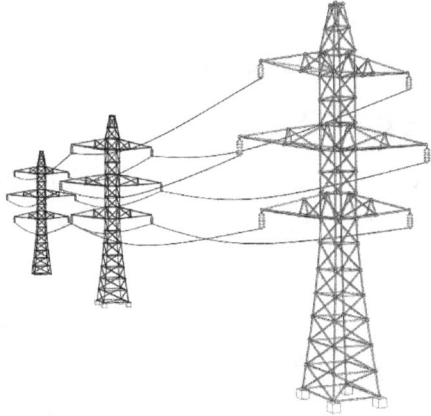

129) **60 Hz sensitivity.** The percentage of people who are hypersensitive to 60 Hz electrical fields is quite small. However, for individuals who are hypersensitive, the typical electrical grid can aggravate the problem, increase health issues, and in some cases, may be the underlying cause of physical health symptoms, although grounding may resolve such symptoms. For some individuals, limited use of electronic devices may be essential. Avoiding living or working in areas of high voltage electrical wires may be an important health consideration for a few people. A very small town or rural location may be preferable or required for health reasons. This is a topic that deserves more study as there is currently a lack of scientific consensus.

Friends or family members, and some health care professionals, may think such problems are emotional or mental health issues, or otherwise downplay these EMF concerns. The reality is that each of us has a unique DNA and sensitivity to various factors in our environment, including electrical fields and other energy influences. The response to EMF fields varies from one person to another.

The science on this is not yet conclusive; however, some public schools and individuals are making an effort to consider high tension stations and transmission lines in an effort to be proactive with regard to the effects of electrical energy fields on the human body.

130) **Vibration.** The effect of extended mechanical vibration is a different kind of energy. Good examples include factories or other work situations, like a jackhammer breaking up concrete, or a commercial rug-cleaning or floor-finishing machine, or smaller homeowners' tools, like an impact hammer, lawnmower, or weed-eater. The direct physical effect on the operator's nerves (intense overstimulation) can cause numbness. For this reason, occupational safety regulations may specify certain work breaks for people using vibrating equipment. Self-employed people and do-it-yourself folks also need to be aware of not overdoing hours of work with vibrating equipment. When you're using such equipment, make an effort to reduce vibration by putting more padding between the equipment and your skin, and be sure to take breaks before your hands get numb.

131)   Crystals. Some kinds of crystals, or those from specific locations, seem to have energetic properties that can be beneficial for some individuals. Whether or not wearing such crystals, or sitting or lying on a pad that has crystals embedded in it, can reduce pain, or improve other aspects of health, appears to vary significantly from one person to another. Before committing significant dollars to a purchase, try anything in this category out for at least several days. They often don't come with guarantees!

132)   Medical electronic devices. Medical devices that are worn on your body or implanted have come a long way since the first hearing aids and early heart pacemakers were developed decades ago. There are numerous wearable devices; they include devices to record your activity level, monitors for blood sugar, muscle stimulators to assist movement and some prosthetic devices, to name just a few. Implanted devices now include not only heart pacemakers, but also pumps that provide controlled release of pain medications, cochlear implants to improve hearing, and many others. They have made life better for millions of people. Wearable and implanted electronic devices may not have any (unintentional) effect on the function of postural muscles, or other functions beyond their intended purpose, but talk with your physician at sufficient length to have all of your questions answered when considering the use of electronic medical devices.

133) **Other subtle energies.** You may not be aware of the effects of other energy fields in your daily environment; fluorescent lights are just one example. Traditional fluorescent lights (straight tubes) emit a subtle flicker, which can create visual stress or other physical symptoms for some people, even when the flicker is not evident to most people. Compact florescent lights (CFLs) may not have this flicker effect.

In our solar system, solar flares produced by our sun have subtle effects on the energy fields of our planet Earth. Psychic energy is a very subtle energy of humans and some animals; most people aren't consciously aware of it. For those who are aware of their own psychic energy or that of other people, it is a very real and meaningful factor in how they perceive and relate to themselves and others. There are other subtle energies that we know about, but do not yet understand, and undoubtedly others that we have not yet recognized. Make an effort to be respectful of others who may be more aware of and sensitive to subtle energy fields.

12. PHYSICAL AIDS AND HEALTH SUPPORTS

Aids for health and mobility: devices, supplements, electrolytes, vitamins, OTC, and "Big Pharma" (medications)

134) Prosthetic devices for movement

135) Canes

136) Walkers

137) Electric scooters

138) Wheelchairs/ electric wheelchairs

139) Sports wheelchairs

140) Nutritional support

141) Water

142) Nutrition: Protein

143) Nutritional supplements

144) Medications

145) Food additives

Most people want to move on their own two legs for as long as they're able to do so. The reality is that you or a loved one may need physical support at some point in time, whether for injury recovery or a longer duration. The important thing to realize is that accepting the use of a support to assist your health or mobility does not make you less of a person. Used appropriately, assistive devices help you to heal faster or to prevent a more dangerous condition. *Insurance companies often cover the cost for those very reasons*. Look at assistive items as helping your health and mobility, not insulting you personally. Various supplements and prescriptions may also improve your present and future abilities, and your enjoyment of daily living.

134) **Prosthetic devices for movement.** From back braces to ankle braces, and from hands to feet, there is a wide world of prosthetic devices to help you perform daily activities better or more easily. Professional health care providers can prescribe these and connect you with trained and skillful technicians. If a prosthetic device goes on your body, wrist, ankle, leg, etc., you must work with special health care professionals—often, orthopedic doctors and a local prosthetic specialist. It is important to get the right device and have it properly fitted, and then to have it adjusted or modified as needed for your maximum comfort and benefit. An appropriate brace may not look cute, but it can reduce further damage to a joint and give you more years of less pain and better movement.

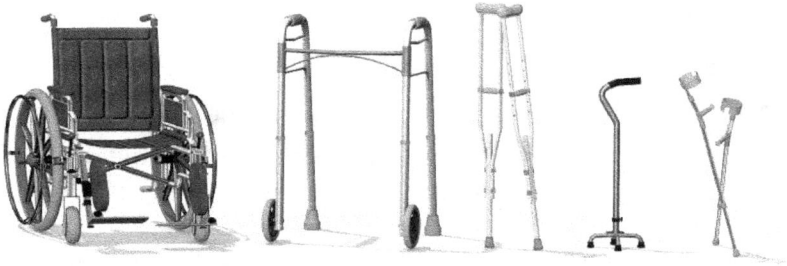

135) **Canes.** If your standing balance is not reliable, a third point of contact with the ground can greatly improve and increase your stability. It can take pressure off a damaged joint or reduce your chance of falling. You can get one without a prescription. There are many varieties of canes, including telescoping ones that can fit easily in a daily tote bag or in a suitcase. Broken bones or a busted head from a fall are far worse than being seen with a cane, especially if your doctor says you need to use a cane. Get one you like and will use. If it's adjustable, be sure someone has adjusted it to the correct height for you. It will be more comfortable and you will be safer using it. Then get over your false pride and inflated ego and just use it!

136) **Walkers.** The same thing goes for walkers as for canes, but more strongly. Using a walker because you're weak or post-operative may not be fun, but at least you're still able to get up and move around more safely. What's worse? Not using it, falling down, and hurting yourself badly enough to be confined to bed, maybe in a hospital? Be glad that you can stand up to use a walker. You might benefit from one that has an option for sitting; many walkers have folding seats so you can sit anytime your feet or legs get tired.

TIP: Be sure someone has adjusted the walker to the correct height for you. It will be more comfortable and you will be safer when using it.

137) **Electric scooters.** Again, like a cane or a walker, look at a mobility aid as a way to enable you to be more independent and able to do some things that your legs, your balance, or your diminished energy will not let you do on foot. A scooter is a way to keep up with others on an outing and an easy way to be less of a burden on others. (They won't have to worry about you falling, and they won't need to be constantly holding your elbow to make sure you have support.) An electric scooter can be a way to accomplish more, or be less fatigued, or both. Embrace this technology if it will make your life better (and yes, you may need to swallow false pride). I can guarantee that you won't be proud of falling down.

138) **Wheelchairs.** If your physical condition requires you to use a wheelchair most or all of the time, you can probably skip this tip because you're probably already under the guidance of a health care professional. If you walk around your house without difficulty, go to the post office or church, or even still drive your own car, you may cringe at the thought of occasionally using a wheelchair or those motorized carts in the airport, *beep-beep-beeping* along with passengers. Let someone with more strength and mobility take responsibility for getting you to the plane on time. You'll feel better when you arrive at your destination. That in itself is a gift of relief to the folks meeting you at your destination.

Do you want to hurt less? Not feel "like such a burden" on family members or friends? Have a big slice of (imaginary) humble pie and take advantage of wheels now and then! You can grocery shop using a motorized chair in the store and still have enough energy afterward to phone friends. Or brag to anyone that you're still able to do your own grocery shopping! Then go take a nice well-earned nap.

Electric wheelchairs. If your personal situation is pointing toward requiring the use of an electric wheelchair, you should be working closely with your local health care providers to determine the characteristics you need in a chair and how you will use and transport it.

139)   Sports wheelchairs. If you're a person who has a competitive streak or a love of physical activity, get out there! Don't let physical challenges put the brakes on your thinking. Use your health care providers, other local contacts, and the internet to explore the range of physical activities and competitive sports that are available for people on wheels. There are financial resources available to help you get a set of wheels appropriate to the activity you want to participate in. Watch scenes from local, state, or Paralympic events to inspire you to get out and move! With purpose and joy in movement, you will be sure to make new friends and maintain or improve your overall health.

140)   Nutritional support. Sometimes the assistance we need is not specifically for mobility; sometimes we need assistance on some aspect of nutrition to help our bodies function better. Your day-to-day food choices can impact your health in ways that you may find very surprising. A lot has been written recently about gluten, gluten sensitivity, and celiac disease. Many people wonder why there is suddenly such a problem for some people eating products made from wheat or other gluten-rich foods. Many of our grandparents and parents ate wheat for years and didn't seem to have these kinds of problems. There is a difference.

Most of the wheat grown commercially in the US today is not the same as the wheat of the 1940s and 1950s. Wheat has been extensively modified (genetically modified organism—GMO) to increase certain qualities. Some changes have been positive (like drought-resistance), but the very large and deliberate increase in the amount of gluten and the type of gluten in wheat has not been good for the human digestive system. Many bakers love certain modern wheat varieties because those varieties contribute to a lighter and fluffier texture in their yeast-raised products. Unfortunately, those same characteristics also make it "sticky" and not as easily digested in our human intestines. These qualities have led many people to realize that at least some of their digestive problems (or other symptoms of poor health) can be reduced by cutting back on foods that contain gluten. Bread and other pastries are on the top of the high-gluten list, but there are many other foods that contain gluten. It is sometimes found in products that you would not expect.

> "The food you eat can be either the safest and most powerful form of medicine or the slowest form of poison."
>
> – Ann Wigmore

TIP: If you have problems with digestion or elimination, consult with a local health care provider who understands nutrition and will take the time to really listen to your concerns and symptoms. There are low-cost ways of finding out if certain foods or food choices are contributing factors to your symptoms.

141)   Water. This nutrient is often underappreciated. Not everyone wants to drink an adequate quantity of plain water, but other beverages, and some foods, also provide fluids that help hydrate your body. Juice, soup, and even tea and coffee provide liquid that your body can utilize for its water needs. Adequate fluid intake is especially important if you suffer from constipation. Often, older people may not be as aware of their thirst and tend to drink less as a result. A lack of adequate fluid in one's daily consumption puts stress on the kidneys and can also be a contributing factor in urinary tract infections.

Dehydration from a lack of fluid consumption can also cause headaches, dizziness, weakness, and impair one's thinking processes. Even for people with mobility issues and people who are concerned about getting to a bathroom soon enough when they feel the urge to go, it is still very important to make a point of consuming enough fluids every day. A generally accepted rule of thumb is to write down your weight in pounds (come on, be honest!) and then divide it by two. Now write "ounces" after that number. That is approximately how much fluid you should be consuming every day. Milk on your cereal counts. Juicy fruits count. Tea and coffee count, sort of; they have some drawbacks and should be only a minor source of your fluid intake. If you sweat or exercise a lot, you'll need more liquids. In (most of) America, we're very fortunate. You do NOT have to buy special water to have clean water to drink and stay hydrated. Just know where the bathrooms are!

142)   Nutrition: Protein. Many Americans get more than enough protein, but others may not. People who are vegetarians, vegans, or raw food proponents may not be getting enough usable protein. People with very limited incomes may not. Senior citizens may also lack adequate protein. Our bodies are less efficient at digesting food as we get older, and many seniors eat smaller quantities of food, and sometimes, less variety. Regardless of your age, your health can suffer when your body is not effective in processing the protein and other nutrients in the food you eat. The immune system can weaken, muscles atrophy (diminish), and hormonal and chemical processes at all levels—from your gut to your skin—can be compromised. Poor health is often the result.

High-quality protein is available in eggs, dairy products, meat, seafood, and certain legumes (beans). If you eat a variety of foods and choose wisely, your brain and your body will thank you. If you're a vegetarian or a vegan, it's important to pay careful attention to be sure you are not cheating your body of essential nutrients, especially vitamin B-12 and well-balanced protein. Soy products are a tempting source of protein, but soy is also high in estrogen, which can upset the hormonal balance in men and women when soy products are used frequently. Soy is added to many prepared foods to raise the protein content, so sometimes people are consuming a much greater amount of soy than they realize. Fiber is also important for digestion, good bowel activity, and regular elimination. Be an informed and conscientious consumer and take your body's needs into account by making the best food choices that you can.

143) **Nutritional supplements.** Countless books have been written on the pros and cons of enhancing your usual food consumption with supplements from a bottle. Without adding to the clamor, here are a few short tips.

a. The Recommended Daily Allowance (RDA) that is included on all vitamin and supplement labels in the US is actually a minimum daily amount that the average adult body needs. Below that level, the body can be deficient and may lack an adequate amount of that nutrient to remain healthy (i.e., to keep from becoming sick). A minimum amount is not exactly the best choice to stay as healthy as you can be. Do you keep a minimum amount of gas in your car? Or a minimum amount of food in your pantry? Or a minimum amount of money in your savings account to keep the bank from closing it? "Better than minimum" is a good investment in your health that will reap positive benefits.

b. If at all possible, consult with a qualified health care provider to find out from routine lab tests where your body is in nutritional terms and what can be done to move toward optimum health. Ask about the best ways for you to work toward those goals.

c. Supplements are available in a wide range of quality; get the best you can reasonably afford. Products certified by an independent laboratory are usually preferred over brands that may (or may not) do their own quality testing or store brands that often make no mention of quality testing at all.

144)   **Medications.** OTC (over-the-counter) products and prescription pharmaceutical products sometimes have a place in our lives. The goal is to not let them become central. Don't use an over-the-counter product to cover up symptoms for weeks or months! That's like putting masking tape over your car's blinking oil light! (Would you really do that?) The real problem can get much worse and cost you much more time and money and health. Some OTC products can be habit-forming and cause withdrawal symptoms—some headache medications, for example, but there are others as well.

Prescription drugs. Many have negative side effects, which may require another prescription! A pharmacist where you get your prescriptions filled can be an excellent source of information on drug interactions and side effects. Pharmacists are highly educated and knowledgeable professionals. Don't hesitate to check with them if you have any questions about either prescriptions or OTC medications that you're using. Also try lifestyle changes. Improvements in your health may be slower, but they are better for you in the long run than depending on pharmaceuticals to override harmful lifestyle choices.

145)   Food additives. Sometimes additives are relatively harmless. You can choose to judge the value and necessity of these additives individually. Added colors are not really necessary; chemical flavors should not be necessary either. Choosing to use fewer commercially processed or prepackaged mixes and products is usually a choice in the direction of better nutrition and better health. Monosodium glutamate, usually known by its abbreviation MSG, is a "flavor enhancer." It occurs naturally in some foods (most notably in seaweed) but usually in very small amounts in other foods. It's added to many prepared foods (such as soups, sauces, and flavoring packets) in the US as a cheap way to boost the perceived flavor. For some people, the quantity in a single serving can be sufficient to act as a neurotoxin (nerve poison), causing headaches, upset stomach, increased heart rate, or other undesirable symptoms.

If you or those you care for have any neurological issues, try to remove MSG from your diet for two or three weeks and see if you observe any improvements. It can be hard to identify MSG on package labels as many manufacturers are using alternative words to get around using the term MSG.

TIP: Avoid additives that do not improve the nutritional value of a food. If you don't know what the ingredient on the label is, buy something else with a short and simple ingredient list.

13. MIND AND BODY (BONUS CHAPTER)

The human body is composed of incredibly complex interwoven systems (as you may have guessed by now!)— not only physically, but mentally, energetically, and also spiritually, however you choose to define that last category. I like to say, "The complexity of the human body makes the international space station look like a prekindergarten project." Our current mainstream/allopathic medical knowledge has only scratched the surface. We all have a lot to learn.

146)   Emotions affect muscles, and vice versa. Identify sources of physical and emotional stress in your life and do whatever you can to reduce causes or levels of stress. Reducing stress can immediately help reduce the frequency and intensity of pain that you experience. Swap childcare duties with a friend; make your workstation more comfortable; take one-minute stretch breaks at least every half hour ... you get the idea. Good choices can contribute to better physical and emotional health because the two are very closely linked.

> "It's not what happens to you, but how you react to it that matters."
>
> – Epictetus

Clinical experience has demonstrated that basic emotions (fear, anger, etc.) significantly affect muscle groups throughout the body, and therefore also affect posture. When processing any event, your brain generates specific physical, emotional, and chemical reactions, which then create predictable muscle responses. For example, when you are angry, muscles are activated to stand tall and confront or fight. If you are scared, muscles are activated for you to crouch low and hide, or maybe run away. Mental health professionals and others also recognize that postures are often related to particular emotional states.

On the flip side of that, the muscles that maintain your typical posture affect your breathing and the chemical/hormonal activity throughout your body all day long. So your muscles affect the physiology (biochemical activity) in your brain, which then affects the way you respond emotionally to everything in your daily life. Physical exercise, mind therapies, and other activities (play, socializing, creative projects, etc.) can therefore all be helpful in changing both your muscle tension and your emotional responses.

147) **Stress and body chemistry.** Engaging regularly in activities that have been shown to reduce the body's stress responses is really helpful. These can include things as simple as a walk, or even just sitting in a natural setting; listening to the calming sounds of music; doing meditation, prayer, yoga or tai chi, etc. It can also include tending plants, spending time with your pet, going for a good run, or enjoying a quiet game of solitaire. The choices are almost endless, and many are free.

Any kind of stress—muscle tension, too little sleep, emotional stress, even a food or an odor that makes your system react—causes your body to release certain stress chemicals (cortisol, adrenaline, and others).

The nerves in your body that are the most hyper-irritated (the ones working overtime to keep overtired muscles stimulated and on the job) are poised on the edge of trouble. Just the slightest increase in physical or emotional tension can push those nerves over the edge ...

and you become (suddenly!) aware of *pain* as they jab your muscles that have been overworked one time too many. Your body responds to those chemical changes in the muscles that have the highest level of neurological stress. Those muscles are typically the first to respond, sending your brain signals of dysfunction or pain. So when you say "stress always goes to my neck" or "my back just went out!" you're quite close to the truth. You have just identified the part of your body that is most chronically tense, and the nerves supplying those muscles or joints as the most hyper-irritated nerves in your musculoskeletal system. Reducing or negating your body's stress-chemical reactions is important.

148) **Breathing.** Here is an immediate stress reducer: use deeper, slower breathing to reduce your body's stress response. When you are confronted with an immediately stressful situation (a spilled drink, an angry person, etc.) first take a very deep, slow breath, then take more deep breaths while you mentally count to 10. And then respond in a voice and with words that you are intentionally trying to keep calm and rational. If you have enough time before a response is required, say a favorite nursery rhyme, a calming prayer, or a short chant to yourself. Such deeply memorized lines can take you emotionally and physically to a place that is more neutral, supportive, and nonthreatening; it will enable you to respond in a less stressful way to any situation.

149) **Laughter.** This has tremendous power to defuse a stressful situation. If you can find non-hurtful humor in the stressful moment, use it. People who are laughing often forget their hurt or angry feelings, at least long enough for a calmer resolution of the situation. Take a deep breath. Spilled milk? "Well, white carpets can be beautiful, but I don't think our fridge could hold enough gallons to turn the whole rug white!"

For longer stress relief, turn to comedies or comedians that you enjoy. Medical researchers have shown that laughter is a stress reducer that actually creates a wide array of beneficial changes in your body. A half hour of good deep belly laughter can release enough endorphins (your body's own morphine-like molecules) to override anxiety or chronic pain for a while and contribute to hours of restorative sleep. Find and enjoy your favorite kind of comedy! It's a very fun way to help your body toward relaxation, better sleep, and better health.

150) **Quieting the mind, body, & spirit.** Make time every day for a quiet period—even just 15 or 20 minutes. The more busy and hectic your days are, the more important it is to create this time. Relaxation response training (developed by Dr. Herbert Benson) and meditation have been researched extensively and their benefits are notable. Meditation in its most basic form is just sitting quietly, relaxed, clearing your mind of the many distractions that can be stressful or overwhelming. It doesn't need to be associated with religious or spiritual beliefs. It takes some practice to learn to meditate or use the "relaxation response" effectively, but the mental and physical rewards are worth it. Regularly quieting your mind has many documented benefits, including lowering blood pressure, reducing cortisol levels, and relieving pain.

Prayer can serve a similar purpose, calming and quieting the mind. By taking your attention to a higher power, expressing gratitude for blessings, or expressing care and concern for others, your mind and body will let go of immediate worries and your stress level can drop significantly. The Roman Catholic saying of the rosary and the other prayers and rituals of many religions are also ways to calm your mind and relax your body. Although not as extensively researched as meditation, the benefits of regular prayer and spiritual practices have been documented. Creating a regular meditative or spiritual time in your daily life will have positive benefits for your mind and body. If you make it the same time every day, it will help create a pattern of restoring your quiet center—a part of your daily routine to care for your mental and physical

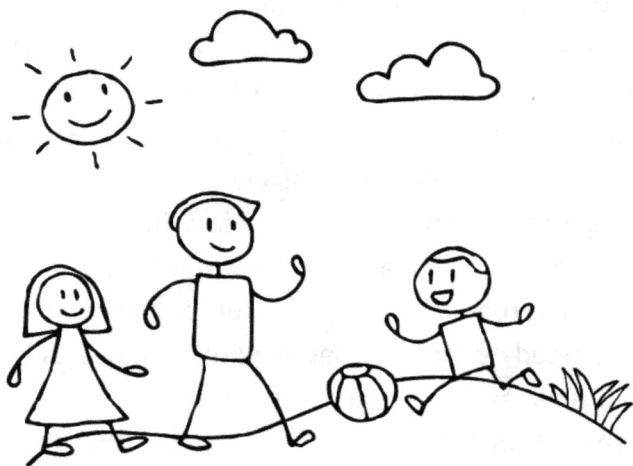

self.

151)   The natural world. Take a walk outdoors if at all possible, preferably where there are plants and trees. The mental and physiological benefits of spending time outdoors, in our natural world, have been studied recently. The health benefits documented thus far include lower blood pressure, blood glucose levels, and stress hormones. Your brain also functions in a better and healthier way. Furthermore, exposure to nature can reduce mental fatigue, respiratory tract and cardiovascular illnesses; improve vitality and mood; benefit issues of mental well-being such as anxiety; and restore attention capacity.

"Forest bathing" is popular in Japan and growing in the US. The soaking isn't literal. This bathing means immersing yourself in the natural environment; intentionally going outside to relax with nature, and allowing nature to help you relax. There are many reasons people are drawn to spend time out of doors in natural environments, walking in parks or on beaches, enjoying forest hikes, or having picnics. Whether it is under sun or clouds, moon or stars, the sky above is a reminder that we live in a natural universe.

> " ... be gentle with yourself. You are a child of the universe, no less than the trees and the stars; you have a right to be here."
>
> –Max Ehrmann, *Desiderata* © 2003

On the physical level, in a place with plants and trees, those living forms release oxygen and take up the carbon dioxide that we exhale; it's a natural exchange of essential elements that benefits both. Modern hospitals are incorporating more windows and garden spaces and making an effort for every patient to have at least a glimpse of nature, as even having a window onto nature has been shown to shorten healing time. Office workers can also benefit from a window, even if they only see a bit of sky.

If you are in a highly urban environment, where manmade structures predominate and a park may not be nearby, consider another option: create a nature space in your home. Play recordings of natural sounds and view images of nature (the larger the better, but your computer screen might have to do). Immerse your senses in natural sounds and images—birds and forests, gardens, sunsets, and star-studded skies—with some frequency. Try to nurture at least one living plant indoors (golden pothos are excellent for this use). And of course, whenever you can, get out into real nature, which offers so much more. (See Chapter 11, Tip #126, for information on the even greater benefits of "grounding" when you're outdoors.)

152) **Calming movement: yoga, tai chi.** Our bodies are meant to move. Contrary to the wishes of some folks, "couch potato" is not a natural position or condition! Some activities like tai chi and yoga can be performed as moving meditations. These provide a combination of physical activity and mental quieting that can be a good fit if you're a person who prefers physical movement over the passive pose of seated meditation or prayer. "Walking meditation" offers a similar option.

Calming movements are a good choice for almost any time of day and can be done by people who are not able or ready for more vigorous exercise. Calmer styles of yoga can be a good choice. They offer a gentle range of motion movements, easier poses, and low-stress "stretching" types of movements that can lead the body toward a better physical condition. Tai chi, sometimes described as a moving meditation, is a standing movement activity in which one shifts gradually and smoothly from one pose to another, with an emphasis on balance and total body coordination from the soles of the feet to the top of the head. Like yoga, it's calming while also providing many benefits for the neuromusculoskeletal system.

153) Take a "news fast." No, this does not mean getting your news quicker by computer, Twitter, or a blog. It means take a BIG break from all news for one week. Give your brain and your body a break from all that tension. A news fast can be very cleansing and calming. Dr. Andrew Weil recommended this back in 1995 in chapter 14 of his book *Spontaneous Healing*; it is so much more needed today. The world will still turn, even if you aren't tuned in for a week. If there's calamitous weather or someone really close to you or important dies, someone will manage to tell you, without you asking.

Too much news, especially if you're bombarding your mind with "the latest!" 16-plus hours a day or more, is really not healthy for your body or your brain. Your continual anticipation of "what's next?" keeps your nervous system amped up. It becomes constantly on alert, which means that your body is stimulated to produce cortisol (and other stress hormones/chemicals) all day long. You're probably not being chased by hungry lions, so you don't need this hyper-awareness! Those physical changes in your body stimulate weight gain, lower your immune response, increase anxiety, and in general create the opposite of a calm mind and good health. When your mind and body are constantly on edge, your personal relationships—at work, at home, and in leisure—may also suffer.

Are you a news addict? Maybe going off news cold turkey isn't for you. If you think that you'll die without constant news for a week, just try it for three or four days. Or limit your news consumption to one hour per day, preferably in the evening (but not just before bedtime). See if you feel or act differently without that nonstop stress all day long. You may be more calm, and the real, live, face-to-face relationships in your world may be better when you give them your undivided attention.

154)   Support groups. Face it. A lot of us have issues that keep us from being and doing our best. Having a group of people with whom you can hash out issues can be very helpful in making your life better. And the fact is that family members or friends who are involved with your emotional baggage are usually not the best ones to help you out of it. Find and join a group that will help you get some heavy or awkward stuff off your chest. It's not weakness to acknowledge a shortcoming; facing uncomfortable truths demonstrates courage and strength.

Support groups exist for almost any problem. Don't believe me? Just check the internet! Concerned you're becoming a hoarder? Are you drinking too much or too often? Is gambling taking over your finances? Do you suffer from depression? Are you addicted to computer gaming 12 hours a day? Or maybe you're suffering from tough medical issues? There are groups for all of these and many more. Some support groups are local and face-to-face interactions (put your town in the search bar); many others exist as online support groups. Other people who are dealing with the same concerns will understand the problems that are challenges for you. They can help because they're also living them. They can offer insights, ideas, and different perspectives, and support you as you work to make positive changes in your life. Pretending that you don't have a problem, or ignoring one that you know you have, doesn't make for a happy or successful life or good relationships. Be that strong person. Dare yourself to grow into a better future.

155)   Grief support/counseling. Too many people think that grief is a solo thing. In reality, all of us will face the loss of someone we love at some point in our lives. It may even be the loss of a very dear pet that tears your heart open. Find a grief support group or counselor. Sharing your loss and your grief can take the edge off the pain. One of my favorite quotes, author unknown, is: "A joy shared is a joy doubled; a trouble shared is half the trouble." You will get ideas on how to get through dark days and darker nights.

If you just ignore your grief, or try to deal with it by yourself, you risk sliding into depression, or becoming stuck in some other aspect of your life. When a loss has hit you hard, don't hesitate to reach out for support. Discuss your agony with others who have suffered a similar loss; learn from each other ways to cope and move on. There are recognized stages of grief; learning what those stages are can help you understand the grief recovery process. Encourage family members or friends who have suffered the same loss to follow your lead toward healing.

156)   Mental health counselors. Many of the comments in the two previous tips apply to seeking the services of a professional in the counseling field. Sometimes a well-trained individual is really what you need to provide a third-party perspective on how to cope with a challenging problem or overcome life experiences that have left you with physical and/or emotional damage. Search out counseling options, then just pick up the phone and make that first call or email.

It can be more affordable—and more beneficial—than you think. If counseling is not covered by your employer or your insurance company, look a little further. One-on-one counseling can be affordable through various service agencies and religious organizations; some counselors are free, and others charge on a sliding scale based on one's income or family resources. The important thing is to make the effort. Improve your ability to view and respond in better ways to the world around you, and many other aspects of your life will also improve. You deserve to have a happier life. Take the necessary steps to help that happen. Why not? People hire coaches every day to improve their performance in sports or their success in business. A mental health counselor is a coach for your personal life.

Mental health counselors usually conduct sessions face to face, but technology is now offering other options via the internet and web cameras. Find someone with whom you feel comfortable, and put your mind and heart into feeling better and functioning more effectively. Acknowledge that you're not perfect (no one is, despite what they say!) and take pride in seeking the benefits that come from working with a good coach to improve your life. The personal rewards are great.

157) **Volunteering.** Of the many ways to make your life better, volunteering may be one of the most interesting and enriching. Bored? Lonely? Want to meet some new people? Look around your neighborhood or community for ways to help other individuals or a cause you support. Need to expand your social circle in a direction more suited to your current needs or interests? Volunteering is a great way to meet other people who are interested in similar things. The opportunities are almost endless. Your computer, local librarians, and civic associations are helpful resources. Besides the intrinsic satisfaction of giving, some volunteer efforts may be rewarded with tickets to events, gift certificates, or other incentives to get out and be of service in your community. Volunteering is a win-win!

FINAL THOUGHTS

In a baker's dozen chapters, I hope you have found some gems of information that you can jump on right away to make your life more pleasant. Take action on the ones that spoke most loudly to you, then come back and try implementing a few other tips.

These ideas may have helped you work toward less pain and better function, but maybe you need something more. When tips are not enough, what's next?

Maybe it's time to seek out a different doctor. If you don't have good two-way communication with your doctor (maybe he or she is your primary care physician), start looking around. Health care professionals have different approaches, different philosophies, and different ways of interacting with their patients, depending on their training and their personality.

Make a genuine effort to find a medical provider with whom you can communicate easily and effectively. It's important to feel that you and your doctor are on the same page. It can make a real difference in the quantity, quality, and variety of information he/she provides. It also impacts how comfortable you are discussing your concerns with that person and the confidence you have in accepting their recommendations.

Doctors who practice functional medicine are becoming more common, and their approach is to look at how different systems of the body work together and affect each other. This wider look is more "whole-person" centered and can offer different insights than single-focus specialists.

If you aren't satisfied with the health care advice you're receiving, you may need to look outside of who (and what) your insurer covers. Whether or not you have insurance, it might be worthwhile to look into different kinds of health care options that you haven't previously considered. "Complementary" modalities—from acupuncture, to nutrition, to physical therapy, to yoga instruction and many others—can offer alternative approaches to improving your mobility, lifestyle habits, and overall health. Educate yourself on a wide range of options so you can make more informed choices. You only have one body, and how you care for it will be reflected in all aspects of your life, for all the years you have left.

Regardless of your age, do whatever you can, in steps large or small, to improve the quality of your life. You're worth it. You won't regret the effort.

This may be the end of this book—

but it's the beginning of better function for you.

REFERENCES

Chapter 1. #1. Shoes (and Socks)

Chapter 1. #9. Rocker-soled Shoes

Klein, M. (2017, May 2). Footwear science: Rocker soles. In Doctors of Running. Retrieved from http://www.doctorsofrunning.com/2017/05/footwear-science-rocker-soles.html.

Chapter 2. #22. Ball-Chairs

https://www.mayoclinic.org/diseases-conditions/back-pain/expert-answers/back-pain-relief/faq-20057793. Accessed March-13-2019.

https://www.prevention.com/fitness/fitness-tips/a20466035/should-you-replace-your-office-chair-with-a-stability-ball/.

Chapter 4. #37. Visual Concerns

Myopia (Nearsightedness) News (n.d.). In HealthDay. Retrieved from https://consumer.healthday.com/eye-care-information-13/myopia-nearsightedness-news-491/Smartphones-summer-birth-could-raise-kids-odds-for-nearsightedness-739426.htm (updated Nov. 7, 2018).

American Academy of Ophthalmology. (2018, August 6). Is too much screen time harming children's vision?

The American Academy of Ophthalmology helps parents separate the facts from fiction. ScienceDaily. Retrieved March 6, 2019 from www.sciencedaily.com/releases/2018/08/1808061627 18.htm.

Heiting, G. (n.d.). Myopia causes – is your child at risk?. In All About Vision. Retrieved from https://www.allaboutvision.com/parents/myopia-causes.htm.

Chapter 4. #48. Constant Sound

Lifewire, Sam Costello. How to Avoid iPhone & iPod Hearing Loss. Updated September 14, 2018. https://www.lifewire.com/tips-to-avoid-iphone-ipod-hearing-loss-1999472.

Martinez, S. J. (2011, December 15). How the iPod and other audio devices are destroying your ears. The Atlantic. Retrieved from https://www.theatlantic.com/health/archive/2011/12/how-the-ipod-and-other-audio-devices-are-destroying-your-ears/249521/.

Audiologist Suggests iPod Users Take Precautions. December 20, 2005 | by Wendy Leopold https://www.northwestern.edu/newscenter/stories/2005/12/garstecki.html.

Noise-induced hearing loss (n.d.). In NICDCD. Retrieved from https://www.nidcd.nih.gov/health/noise-induced-hearing-loss. Last updated Feb 7, 2017.

Chapter 9. #103. Kids and Sports

King's College London. "Genetic differences may influence sensitivity to pain, according to new study." ScienceDaily. ScienceDaily, 20 December 2012. www.sciencedaily.com/releases/2012/12/1212201718 10.htm.

"American genes." ScienceDaily. ScienceDaily, 20 April 2014. <www.sciencedaily Academy of Neurology (AAN). "Low tolerance for pain? The reason may be in your.com/releases/2014/04/140420193428.htm>.

Chapter 9. #105. Concussions

Elsevier. (2018, August 14). Study identifies distinct origin of ADHD in children with history of brain injury. ScienceDaily. Retrieved March 6, 2019 from www.sciencedaily.com/releases/2018/08/1808141013 02.htm.

Mastroianni, B. (2018, April 17). Research suggests that kids with brain injuries have a higher risk of ADHD. In *Everyday Health*. Retrieved from https://www.everydayhealth.com/neurology/sympto ms/research-suggests-kids-with-brain-injuries-have-higher-risk-adhd.

Traumatic brain injury in children can lead to ADHD years later. Megan Narad. JAMA Pediatrics. March 19, 2018. https://www.healthline.com/health-news/ traumatic-brain-injury-in-children-lead-to-adhd.

The association between traumatic brain injury and ADHD in a Canadian adult sample, Gabriela Ilie et al., Journal of Psychiatric Research, DOI: http://dx.doi.org/10.1016/j.jpsychires.2015.08.004, published online 7 August 2015, abstract.

Chapter 9. #106. Yoga & Tai chi

Peter M. Wayne, Douglas P. Kiel, and David E. Krebs, et al.. The Effects of Tai Chi on Bone Mineral Density in Postmenopausal Women: A Systematic Review.. Archives of Physical Medicine and Rehabilitation. 2007. DOI: https://doi.org/10.1016/j.apmr.2007.02.012.

Zou, L., Wang, C., Chen, K., Shu, Y., Chen, X., Luo, L., & Zhao, X. (2017). The effect of taichi practice on attenuating bone mineral density loss: A systematic review and meta-analysis of randomized controlled trials. International Journal of Environmental Research and Public Health, 14(9), 1000. doi:10.3390/ijerph14091000.

Chapter 11. #128. Earth's negative ion field

Earthing: The Most Important Health Discovery Ever! (2014) Ober, Sinatra, & Zucker. Basic Health Publications, Inc.; 2nd ed. (March 15, 2014) Paperback: 338 pages. ISBN-13: 978-1591203742.

Chevalier, G. & Mori, K. The effect of earthing on human physiology (part II): Electrodermal measurements. Subtle Energy and Energy Medicine, (2007): 18(3): 11-34.

Chapter 11. #129. 60 Hz sensitivity

Energy Medicine: The Scientific Basis. (2000). James L. Oshman. Churchill Livingstone; 1st edition (May 29, 2000). Paperback: 296 pages. ISBN-10: 0443062617. ISBN-13: 978-0443062612.

Chapter 12. #140. Nutritional support (boxed quote)

Ann Wigmore. https://www.goodreads.com/quotes/563016-the-food-you-eat-can-be-either-the-safest-and.

Wigmore, Ann. The Wheatgrass Book: How to Grow and Use Wheatgrass to Maximize Your Health & Vitality. Avery; 1st edition 1985. 144 pages.

Chapter 13. #146. Emotions affect muscles, and vice versa (boxed quote)

Epictetus. https://www.brainyquote.com/topics/react
.

Chapter 13. #149. Laughter

Head First: The biology of hope. Norman Cousins. (1989). Dutton; 1st edition (1989). Hardcover: 368 pages. ISBN-10: 0525248056. ISBN-13: 978-0525248057 (Chapter 10: The Laughter Connection, pp 125 - 153).

Chapter 13. #150. Quieting the Mind & Spirit.

Relaxation Revolution: The Science and Genetics of Mind Body Healing. Benson & Proctor. Scribner; 1st edition (June 21, 2011). Paperback: 288 pages. ISBN-10: 143914866X; ISBN-13: 978-1439148662.

Spontaneous Healing. Andrew Weil. Fawcett Columbine (2000). (Chapter 13: Mind, Body, Spirit). Paperback: 376 pages. ISBN-10: 0804117942. ISBN-13: 978-0804117944. ASIN: B0073XT67U.

"Desiderata." Max Ehrmann. Scholastic Press; 1st edition (March 1, 2003). ISBN-10: 9780439372930. ISBN-13: 978-0439372930. ASIN: 0439372933.

Chapter 13. #151. Natural world

How might contact with nature promote human health? Promising mechanisms and a possible central pathway. *Frontiers in Psychology*, 2015; 6 DOI: 10.3389/fpsyg.2015.01093

University of East Anglia. "It's official – spending time outside is good for you." ScienceDaily. ScienceDaily, 6 July 2018. www.sciencedaily.com/releases/2018/07/180706102842.htm.

Williams, F. (2017, June 7). This is your brain on nature. *National Geographic*. Retrieved from https://www.nationalgeographic.com/magazine/2016/01/call-to-wild/.

BBC – "Earth: How nature is good for our health and happiness" Apr 20, 2016. Dr Richardson.

www.bbc.com/earth/story/20160420-how-nature-is-good-for-our-health-and-happiness.

Lauren F. Friedman and Kevin Loria. "11 scientific reasons you should be spending more time outside." Business Insider, *Business Insider*, 22 Apr. 2016.

Haile, Rahawa. "'Forest Bathing': How microdosing on nature can help with stress." *The Atlantic*, Atlantic Media Company, 30 June 2017.

Taylor AF, Kuo FE. Children with attention deficits concentrate better after walk in the park. J Atten Disord. 2009;12(5):402-9.

How Hospital Gardens Help Patients Heal. *Scientific American* (March 2012), 306, 24-25. Published online: 14 February 2012 | doi:10.1038/scientificamerican0312-24.

Chapter 13. #153. Take a "news fast"

Spontaneous Healing. Andrew Weil. (2000). Ballantine Books. (Chapter 14. pp. 262-272) 384 page. ISBN-10: 9780804117944. ISBN-13: 978-0804117944. ASIN: 0804117942.

Heid, M. (2018, January 31). You asked: Is it bad for you to read the news constantly? Time. Retrieved from http://time.com/5125894/is-reading-news-bad-for-you/.

Traumatic events in the news causes spikes in stress (2015, November 10). In Anxiety.org. Retrieved from https://www.anxiety.org/news-increases-stress.

"ASK DR. FLO"

ABOUT THE AUTHOR

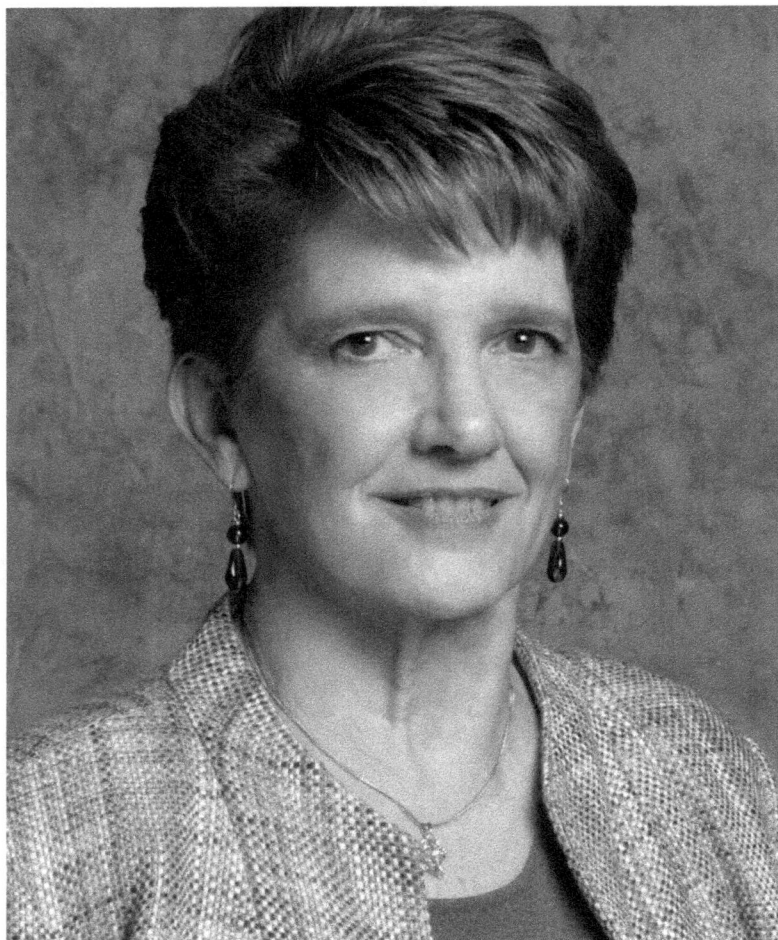

Flo Barber-Hancock, LMT, Ph.D, has been a health care provider in Tampa, Florida, for over 20 years at Hancock Holistic Clinic. She is a pioneer in the development of CranioSomatic Therapy with her husband, Dr. G. Dallas Hancock. Her clinical internship with him in the mid-1990s provided a strong grounding in evaluating neurosensory and motor dysfunctions. That experience led her to develop an innovative manual therapy (Facilitated Pathways Intervention) for neuromusculoskeletal dysfunctions; it became the subject of her Ph.D. in Neurosensory Rehabilitation. She and her husband teach their concepts and techniques in the US and internationally through Hancock CranioSomatic Institute.

Dr. Flo treats patients of all ages who have joint or muscle pain, difficulties with movements, or sensory dysfunctions. Her insights into how routine activities and daily movements can create or perpetuate discomfort led to numerous tips for her patients. Now you can benefit from these 150 tips!

Visit www.HancockClinic.com
or www.CranioSomatics.com to keep up with Dr. Flo.

Website: www.FloBarber.com
www.CranioSomatics.com
Email: floBarber@CranioSomatics.com

Address inquiries to:
Flo Barber-Hancock, LMT, Ph.D.
Hancock CranioSomatic Institute
7827 N. Armenia Ave.
Tampa, Florida 33604
Phone: 813-933-6335
USA Toll-free: 888-824-7025